# SANCTUARY

## The Inner Life of Home

Edited by Valerie Andrews

CHIRON PUBLICATIONS • ASHEVILLE, NORTH CAROLINA

© 2024 by Chiron Publications. All rights reserved. No part of this publication may be reproduced, stored in a retrieval system, or transmitted, in any form by any means, electronic, mechanical, photocopying, recording, or otherwise, without the prior written permission of the publisher, Chiron Publications, P.O. Box 19690, Asheville, N.C. 28815-1690.

www.ChironPublications.com

Interior and cover design by Danijela Mijailovic

Printed primarily in the United States of America.

Cover image - Section of *A Room in the Artist's Home in Strandgade, Copenhagen, with the Artist's Wife,* Vilhelm Hammershøi, Public Domain

Author photo on back cover by Boris Zharkov

ISBN 978-1-68503-217-3 paperback
ISBN 978-1-68503-218-0 hardcover
ISBN 978-1-68503-219-7 electronic
ISBN 978-1-68503-220-3 limited edition paperback


Library of Congress Cataloging-in-Publication Data Pending

# Acknowledgements

I would like to thank my friend and colleague, Jean Shinoda Bolen, for supporting this book and for serving on the advisory board of *Reinventing Home*, an experiment in non-profit journalism that considered the vast changes in our domestic lives during and after the pandemic.

Each contributor to this volume has amplified our understanding of our age-old quest for home and our need for a deep sense of belonging. I'm grateful to these writers from many different disciplines for showing why home is essential is to our health and wellbeing. Special thanks to Phil Cousineau, who translated the poem by Marie Noel in the Introduction ("Our houses are learning/Not to be so careful and so cautious") and told me about the French artist Vincent Adelus, who has made his home into a work of art with illuminated images in every window. For endless conversations about the meaning of home, I'm grateful to Phil and to my colleagues at *Reinventing Home*, Ann Arnold and Sara Evans. Additional support came from members of my writers' circle: Mary Reynolds Thompson, Bruce Thompson, and Ann Robinson. And also, from my women's group: Isabel Allende, Jean Bolen, Grace Dammann, Carole Robinson, and Pauline Tesler. In addition, I would like to acknowledge the superb design and editorial team at Chiron, and its visionary publisher, Dr. Steven Buser, for sending these ideas out into the world and making them available to a broad and receptive audience.

A bow of appreciation to my partner, Russ McClure, who shares my deep sense of home and has supported my years of work on this theme. Finally, this book is dedicated to all those searching for sanctuary in uncertain times.

CONTENTS

# INTRODUCTION
## Our Story of Home

If you want to get to know someone, listen to their story of home. Intimacy builds as we consider the answers to these questions: Where do you come from? What did you leave behind? Who do you long for? Where do you feel safe?

In *Sanctuary*, these themes are explored from an evolutionary psychology perspective by experts in psychology, architecture, history, science, and literature who carry Swiss psychiatrist C.G. Jung's ideas out into the culture. This interdisciplinary approach to home is timely. Since the 2019 coronavirus pandemic, we have pushed our dwellings to the limit, holding endless work meetings on Zoom, homeschooling our children, and caring for vulnerable family members under the same roof. Our sense of home has also been changing on a macro-level. With the social movement Black Lives Matter, and new efforts toward diversity and inclusion, we're reshaping our communities and reconsidering our notion of a just society. At the same time, we're facing the mounting toll of climate change as we rebuild our homes in the wake of fires, floods, and hurricanes. Finally, an unprecedented wave of global refugees is forcing those of us who live in developed nations to re-examine our long-held notions of home and hospitality.

In 2019, I launched a non-profit digital magazine, *Reinventing Home*, to consider how home shapes our culture and our character. The majority of these essays first appeared in that publication. The theme of sanctuary emerged as I began to reflect upon the significance of Jung's retreat at Bollingen, his home on the shore of Lake Zurich. When San Francisco analyst Elizabeth Osterman visited Jung there in 1958, she met a strong-bodied, white-haired 83-year-old in a green workman's apron, chopping wood. "I felt as though I had stepped out of time and entered into an inner world where everything was relevant, unhurried, natural," Osterman wrote.

"I have found the way to live here as part of nature, to live in my own time," Jung told her. "People are always living as if something better is to happen … They are up in the head and don't think to live their lives!"[1] And here is our notion of home as a refuge—and an antidote to the speed and stress of the modern world.

For Jung, the more primitive the setting the better. "I have done without electricity, and tend the fireplace and stove myself," he explained in his autobiography, *Memories, Dreams, Reflections.* "Evenings, I light the old lamps … I pump the water from the well. I chop the wood and cook the food. These simple acts make man simple, and how difficult it is to be simple!"[2] Jung felt that basic domestic tasks—from cooking, cleaning, and gardening to mending walls and splitting wood—have an important psychological function. Simply put, they connect us to our ancestors, and to the flow of life.

Jung likens the psyche to a mansion with many rooms and draws on this as a model for evolutionary psychology. He describes how this structure came to him in a dream:

I was in a house I did not know, which had two storeys. It was "my house." I found myself in the upper storey, where there was a kind of salon furnished with fine old pieces in Rococo style. On the walls hung a number of precious old paintings. I wondered that this should be my house and thought "not bad." But then it occurred to me that I did not know what the lower floor looked like. Descending the stairs, I reached the ground floor. There everything was much older. I realised that this part of the house must date from about the fifteenth or sixteenth century. The furnishings were mediaeval, the floors were of red brick. Everywhere it was rather dark. I went from one room to another, thinking, "Now I really must explore the whole house." I came upon a heavy door, and opened it. Beyond it, I discovered a stone stairway that led down into the cellar. Descending again, I found myself in a beautifully vaulted room which looked exceedingly ancient. Examining the walls, I discovered layers of brick among the ordinary stone blocks, and chips of brick in the mortar. As soon as I saw this I knew that the walls dated from Roman times. My interest by now was intense. I looked more closely at the floor.

It was of stone slabs, and in one of these I discovered a ring. When I pulled it, the stone slab lifted, and again I saw a stairway of narrow stone steps leading down to the depths. These, too, I descended, and entered a low cave cut into rock. Thick dust lay on the floor, and in the dust were scattered bones and broken pottery, like remains of a primitive culture. I discovered two human skulls, obviously very old, and half disintegrated. Then I awoke.[3]

For Jung, home provides a map of our collective evolution and a description of the individual psyche. The salon, or upper level, represents the face one presents to the world. The lower level represents the ideas we inherit from our ancestors and the culture. The basement, the vault, and the cave, contain more primitive states of being—our unconscious urges, dreams, and desires—the raw emotions of which we have little awareness, and even less control. It can be argued that Sigmund Freud's model of the psyche was hydraulic with sexuality as the driving force, while Jung's was architectural with rooms and stairwells leading to different states of consciousness.

Since then, we've had other contributions to the inner life of home. Clare Cooper Marcus, a professor of architecture at UC Berkeley, has explored the house as a mirror of the self. Today, designers like to talk about the way our rooms reflect our personalities. I have found that each portion of my house embodies a different psychological function: the kitchen honors sensation; the bedroom is a place for dreams and intuition; the office is a room for thinking and planning;

and the living room, animated by lively conversation, is guided by the feeling function.

Our inner lives are also shaped by what we see outside the window. The novelist Laurence Durrell observed that all landscapes ask the same question: I am watching you. Are you watching yourself in me?[4] A view of trees or water has an impact on the psyche, as does the layout of our streets and towns. In the 1960s, developers did away with Main Street to construct a morass of malls, fast-food joints, and parking lots, and our communities lost their character. The *New York Times* architecture critic Ada Louise Huxtable summed up our loss of place in a column titled, *Hello Hamburger, Goodbye History*, and in *City and Soul*, James Hillman reminded us how our emotions are affected by our buildings, our neighborhood's walkability, and our access to natural beauty.

For America's founding fathers, home was meant to be a sanctuary, a place where each man had the right to "life, liberty and the pursuit of happiness." But what becomes of these ideals in an age that's dominated by productivity and commerce? Until the coronavirus pandemic, Americans spent more hours at the office than any other developed nation, outperforming the Japanese who invented the word (karoshi) for "death by overwork." Add to that the stress of long commutes and the fact that technology has made us reachable 24/7 and you have the recipe for burnout. With the arrival of COVID-19, we experienced a new kind of stress. In addition to working in isolation, we had to contend with supply chain meltdowns, product shortages, financial uncertainty, and growing political unrest. As I write, the world is wildly tilting with a marked increase in violence, from public shootings to war and civil unrest. Our minds turn once again to our need for sanctuary.

What kind of solace can home offer? In *Honey for a Child's Heart: The Imaginative Use of Books in Family Life*, Gladys Hunt reminds us that home should provide a safe haven. "My favorite definition of home a safe place where one is free from attack, a place where one experiences secure relationships and affirmation," she writes. "It is a place where people share and understand each other. Its relationships are nurturing. The people in it do not need to be perfect; instead, they need to be honest, loving, supportive, recognizing a common humanity that makes all of us vulnerable."[5]

Sanctuary is essential for our overall health and wellbeing according to medical researchers.[6] After analyzing mounds of data, the Centers for Disease Control and Prevention and Kaiser Permanente found that children who come from an unstable home experience a higher rate of depression, alcoholism, diabetes, lung disease, heart attacks, and obesity in adulthood. We now understand that there are profound consequences, for both the individual and society, when our early home life fails to provide us with a proper refuge.

In *The Architecture of Happiness,* Alain de Botton describes home as a shell that protects us from the pressures of the outside world. "We need a home in the psychological sense as much as we need one in the physical," he observes, "to compensate for a vulnerability. We need a refuge to shore up our states of mind because so much of the world is opposed to our allegiances. We need our rooms to align us to desirable versions of ourselves and to keep alive the important, evanescent sides of us."[7]

When a sense of security is lacking, we often try to fix things with a quick renovation. "We depend on our surroundings obliquely to embody the moods and ideas we respect and then to remind us of them," says Botton, "We look to our buildings to hold us, like a kind of psychological mold, to a helpful vision of ourselves. We arrange around us material forms which communicate to us what we need—but are at constant risk of forgetting what we need—within. We turn to wallpaper, benches, (and) paintings … to staunch the disappearance of our true selves."[8]

Our obsession with the Home and Garden Television channel (HGTV), design magazines, and home décor, are symptoms of this loss of soul—and an indication that we need to look at what home means to us on a deeper level.

Jung believed that one day Americans would have to step back from their obsession with commerce and productivity to consider the value of the inner life. As we sheltered in place during the pandemic, we did just that. Many of us pulled back from our workaholic orientation and discovered the benefits of time at home. The result was The Great Resignation, a mass quitting likened by some economists to a general strike. In an interview with the *New York Sun* in the 1930s, Jung noted that that at some point, Americans would have to say no to their conventional drives and expectations:

> What America needs in the face of the tremendous urge toward uniformity, desire of things, the desire for complications in life, for being like one's neighbors … is one great healthy ability to say No, to rest a minute and realize that many of the things being sought

are unnecessary to a happy life … We want simplicity. We are suffering in our cities, from a need to simplify things. We would like to see our great terminals deserted, the streets deserted, a great peace descend upon us.[9]

Our landscape in the early days of the pandemic revealed hushed streets, empty train stations, and abandoned office buildings. At that point, many of us tuned out, and turned our backs on the drive for perfection, productivity, and success. In short, we began to appreciate the solace of the home.

At the close of the 19th century, the German sociologist Max Weber described our need for creature comforts: "Culture will come when every man will know how to address himself to the inanimate simple things of life, when people feel at one with their surroundings, when they are able to "touch things with love and see them with a penetrating eye."[10]

Home is a place we tend to our longings and belongings—it's where we discover that all things want to be cared for and acknowledged. This description of caring for the home brings us to what philosopher Martin Buber called an I-Thou relationship, where we honor our surroundings and cultivate a deep respect for the material world.

A regard for household objects plays a strong role in Jungian lore, as well. Jung enjoyed making simple, hearty meals at his lake house in Bollingen and had a special fondness for his pots and pans. In his later years, he was confined to bed after a serious illness. One morning, he awoke to a loud clanging. Jung immediately knew what was wrong. He put on his slippers and walked into the kitchen and spoke to his pots, essentially telling them, "I'll be back with you soon, and we'll make some good things together." With that the banging stopped.[11]

While Jung conversed with his possessions, and treated them with kindness, he also acknowledged the shadow side of their behavior. During a seminar in Ascona, Switzerland, Jung described how material things rebel when they feel mistreated or neglected. Jung referred to "die tücke des objekts" (the malice of objects), noting, for example, that a book dislikes being placed on the edge of a table, and that our glasses object to being left haphazardly on a chair. Possessions have much to teach us about our sentience in an age that's soon to be dominated by robots and artificial intelligence.

The question we keep coming back to is this: How can home help us remember what it means to be human? And how can it help us nurture the best and truest version of ourselves? The premise of this book is that home serves as an inner sanctum, a place apart from the collective where we can listen to the promptings of the soul. Jung knew this. That's why he carved this saying in the doorway of his home, "Called or not, the god is present." And it's why he enjoyed reminding visitors of the "little household gods," from the lares and penates the Romans kept on their dining tables to the household spirits celebrated in European folklore.

At midlife, Jung had two houses, each representing a different part of his personality. The grand one in Küsnacht, shared with his wife, Emma and their children, had handsome furniture, stained glass windows, and rich carpets that reflected his growing stature as a physician and psychiatrist. In this airy, spacious place, he received his patients and colleagues in his role as the doctor, the problem-solver, and idea-man. On a lake some 20 miles southwest was his retreat at Bollingen where he communed with a much older sense of self. Jung built much of this place by hand, using local stone and tools from the Middle Ages. The house was isolated, primitive. This is where Jung withdrew after his break with Freud, and again, following the death of his wife. Its most remarkable element is the tower Jung added to the building as he entered old age.

"From the beginning," Jung wrote: "I felt the Tower was in some way a place of maturation ... in which I could become what I was, what I am and will be." To the last, it remained a deeply private place, providing Jung with a place to incubate his own memories, dreams, and reflections, helping him to attain a sense of peace. At Bollingen, for part of every year surviving without heat, electricity, or running water, Jung said, "I am in the midst of my true life. I am most deeply myself."[12]

This is Jung speaking toward the end of his career. By now, he has moved from the House of Achievement to the House of Eternity, where he cares more about the fate of the world than his own ambition and accomplishments. Jung is writing from the perspective of that second house when he says:

> We rush impetuously into novelty, driven by a mounting sense of insufficiency, dissatisfaction, and restlessness. We no longer live on what we have, but on promises ... We refuse to recognize that everything better is purchased at the price of something worse ... new methods or gadgets, are of course impressive at first, but in the long run they are dubious and ... dearly paid for.

They, by no means, increase the contentment or happiness of people on the whole. Mostly they are deceptive sweetenings of existence, like speedier communications which unpleasantly accelerate the tempo of life and leave us with less time than ever before.[13]

Modern life, Jung felt, was a distraction from the house that we were all meant to build—the house of reflection, on the shores of a secluded lake.

Artists and writers are also finding new ways to honor the special character of the home. The French poet Marie Noël, nominated for the Nobel Prize in literature, in 1960, believed that the house itself can be a benevolent force, making us feel both whole and holy. In this verse, newly translated by Phil Cousineau, she notes that houses can enfold us in a protective embrace and shield us from the dangers of the outside world. Here she describes a row of homes by the side of the road, filled with good intentions:

> *The houses are learning tonight*
> *To not be so careful and cautious,*
> *So near to the dark road.*
> *You will be far happier about it.*[14]

There are many ways to acknowledge the spirit of a house. When artist Vincent Adelus moved into a new building in Saint-Mihiel, France, he invited a group of friends to make paintings to fill its many tall windows. When passersby look up, they do not encounter a dark façade. Instead, they find a symphony of color—the house as a living, breathing thing.

This is what I hope *Sanctuary* will do for you: Illuminate the spirit of home—and remind you that each dwelling is much richer, and more complex, than it first appears.

In Part I, Home as a Safe Haven considers the various ways we find solace and security within four walls. In "The Poetry of Place," critic Frank Beck considers the role of home in modern literature, and as an anchor in the writer's life. In "Typology at Home" psychological counselor Sally Keil recounts how an understanding of Jung's personality types helped her respond to the needs of her new husband and three stepchildren, creating a sense of sanctuary for them all. In "The Myth of the Man Cave," architect Anthony Lawlor explains why men have always needed a room that allows them to burrow into the unconscious and retreat from the demands of the outside world. Analyst Gilda Frantz takes a novel approach to releasing the energy of other people's things in "Renovating with a Shaman." Frantz describes her difficulty getting rid of boxes she has stored after the deaths of family members and the process of reclaiming her own space. In "Far from the Irish Sea," analyst John Hill describes his memories of home during a serious childhood illness, and the inward journey that took him to the mountains of Switzerland and eventually to a retreat on the isle of Patmos. This portion of the book shows how home provides solace and stability at life's major turning points.

Part II, Home in Times of Trauma, explores how our sense of home is torn apart by war and conflict. In "American Icarus," Pythia Peay describes a growing up with a father who flew for the Air Transport Command in Brazil during World War II, then with Pan Am, and raged at being penned down on a Missouri farm. Peay explores a familiar archetype—the hero who flew too high and had trouble coming down to earth.

In "These Wilds Beyond Our Fences," psychologist Bayo Akomolafe recounts fleeing his house after being held at gunpoint by rebel soldiers in Zaire. His writes a poignant letter to his daughter about the challenges of finding a home in a world full of violence and civil unrest.

In "The Dance of Exile," Biljiana Lipič recounts losing her home and family to a brutal conflict in Sarajevo, eventually finding sanctuary in Jungian psychology and bodywork while living in a houseboat community in Cornwall.

Social worker Andrea Plate provides a stark portrait of daily life at a residence operated by the Veteran's Administration in downtown Los Angeles in "Coming Home to the V.A." Soldiers returning from Viet Nam and Iraq often suffer from multiple addictions, depression, post traumatic stress disorder, and homelessness. Plate raises the important question: How can we expect men and women to fight for American values if we fail to offer them sanctuary when they return?

The final essay in this section deals with another kind of trauma—the threat of illness and disease. For "Pandemic Dreams–Horrors or Healers?" I interviewed Jungians about the disturbing nightmares reported during COVID. At one point, our dreams shifted from a "fight or flight" response to images of hope and regeneration. This chapter shows how a somatic approach to dreaming can help calm the nervous system and allow us to feel at home within our bodies, as well as within the body of the world.

Part III, A New Story of Home considers our need for a new narrative that moves beyond the quest for dominance and power. As analyst Thomas Singer observes in "What Myth Now?" we have been through "a brutal, emotionally draining election cycle accompanied by a pandemic, economic collapse, ever-deepening division, racial violence, floods, and wildfires that have felt apocalyptic." Here he notes:

> "Americans have been in a state of great distress, wondering what the future will hold—yearning for a vision, new or old, that will help resolve what I term 'cultural complexes' that divide us on issues of immigration, race, gender, abortion, health care, the relationship between rural and urban populations, between the individual and the broader community, and our views on the role of government today. If we are serious about engaging the deeper meanings of our individual and collective lives, it is often best to begin at home by asking probing questions. Who am I as a person? Who are we as a people? Where is our country headed?"

Singer considers one possibility—a story based on the ecological model and the interdependence of all living things.

This section of the book focuses on finding our home in the natural world. In "From Active Imagination to Wildlife Preservation," psychologist Andrea Wells tells how she began to dialogue with tortoises and whales that often appeared in her dreams. Over the years, this dialogue led her to volunteer to save these creatures from extinction and also to protect the habitats of rhinos and elephants. Her story is an eloquent reminder that "in dreams begin responsibilities" and that animals, too, need sanctuary.

Another important contribution on this theme is "Grassland Woman: Understanding Nature's Archetypes." In her books and workshops, Mary Reynolds Thompson links the stages of a woman's psychological growth to five landscapes: the Desert, Mountains, Oceans and Rivers, Forests, and Grasslands. Using the framework of archetypal psychology, she makes an eloquent plea for the rewilding of the feminine soul.

Where else are we in need of a new story? The Black Lives Matter movement is calling our attention to issues of equality, and to a population that's been brutally disenfranchised. In "Dialogue on the Mall," Pulitzer Prize-winning author Joseph J. Ellis applies Jung's concept of active imagination to history, conjuring up a conversation with Thomas Jefferson, Abraham Lincoln, and Martin Luther King on the topic of civil rights, asking what it means to protect the home, safety, and a sense of dignity of all Americans.

In the final essay in this section, "Why Activists Need Home," analyst Jean Shinoda Bolen considers the rise of feminism and the importance of home as a place for activists to recharge and regroup. Drawing on her work on the Greek Goddesses, Bolen provides a meditation on the values of Hestia and the comforts of the hearth.

Part IV, Homely Conversations presents five dialogues that center around our experience of longing and belonging. In "Make Your Life Like Music," analyst Helen Marlo describes the plight of working mothers with endless demands on their energy and time. With children, the tempo of the household changes, but keeping up isn't a matter of being better organized. It's about learning how to improvise. Marlo founded the organization Mentoring Mothers to help women explore their early memories of home and consider the kind of home they wish to create for the next generation.

In "Aging at Home," Peggy Flynn considers our history of caring for the sick and dying at home, and how well we manage these responsibilities. Home is the final stage set in the unfolding drama of our lives. As founder of The Good Death Institute, Flynn tells how to organize that stage set according to Maslow's hierarchy of needs. Trained in Jungian psychology, Flynn is sensitive to her clients' typology, and to the many ways that home reflects their core identity. As Jung noted, "The afternoon of life is just as full of meaning as the morning; only, its meaning and purpose are different"[15] Flynn shows how a house must change and grow, along with the psyche, as we enter this final period of life.

In "The Art of Living in Uncertain Times," analyst James Hollis addresses our increasing disorientation in the face of global warming, political unrest, and a volatile economy. In this conversation, Hollis considers how great writers from Sophocles to Shakespeare help us navigate unexpected twists of fate, and why it's important to hold on to our inner sense of home.

In "Homecoming from Homer to The Wizard of Oz," Emmy award-winning writer, filmmaker, and storyteller Phil Cousineau explains our longing for the hearth. Drawing on Western mythology, he zeroes in on the crucial moment at the end of the hero's journey, making sense of all of the adventures, and finally, finding his way home. Cousineau explains why Americans feel so unrooted, and how art, sports, music, and memory can anchor us in a given place.

It seems fitting to end with physicist Brian Swimme's meditation on "Finding Our Home in the Cosmos." With insights from psychology, anthropology, and the sciences, Swimme explains that the universe is engaged in an act of continuous recreation—a process that is reflected in our bodies and our psyches. When our ancestors first looked up at the night sky, they felt this resonance and knew they were part of something vast and mysterious—and that the universe itself was home. Today scientists tell us we are made of the same stuff as the stars. Swimme invokes a sense of awe and wonder as he describes the birth of our galaxy, reminding us that our home address includes the Milky Way.

Futurists predict that we will soon outgrow this planet and begin to colonize another, but the key to living anywhere comes back to the care and tending of the home. "I always wondered why the makers leave housekeeping and cooking out of their tales," Ursula Le Guin says in her science fiction novel *Voices,* "Isn't it what all the great wars and battles are fought for—so that at day's end a family may eat together in a peaceful house?"

No matter how far we travel—to another city or a distant galaxy—we will always be searching for sanctuary, stitching it together from some combination of memory, imagination, and desire.

Valerie Andrews
Mill Valley, California
November 2023

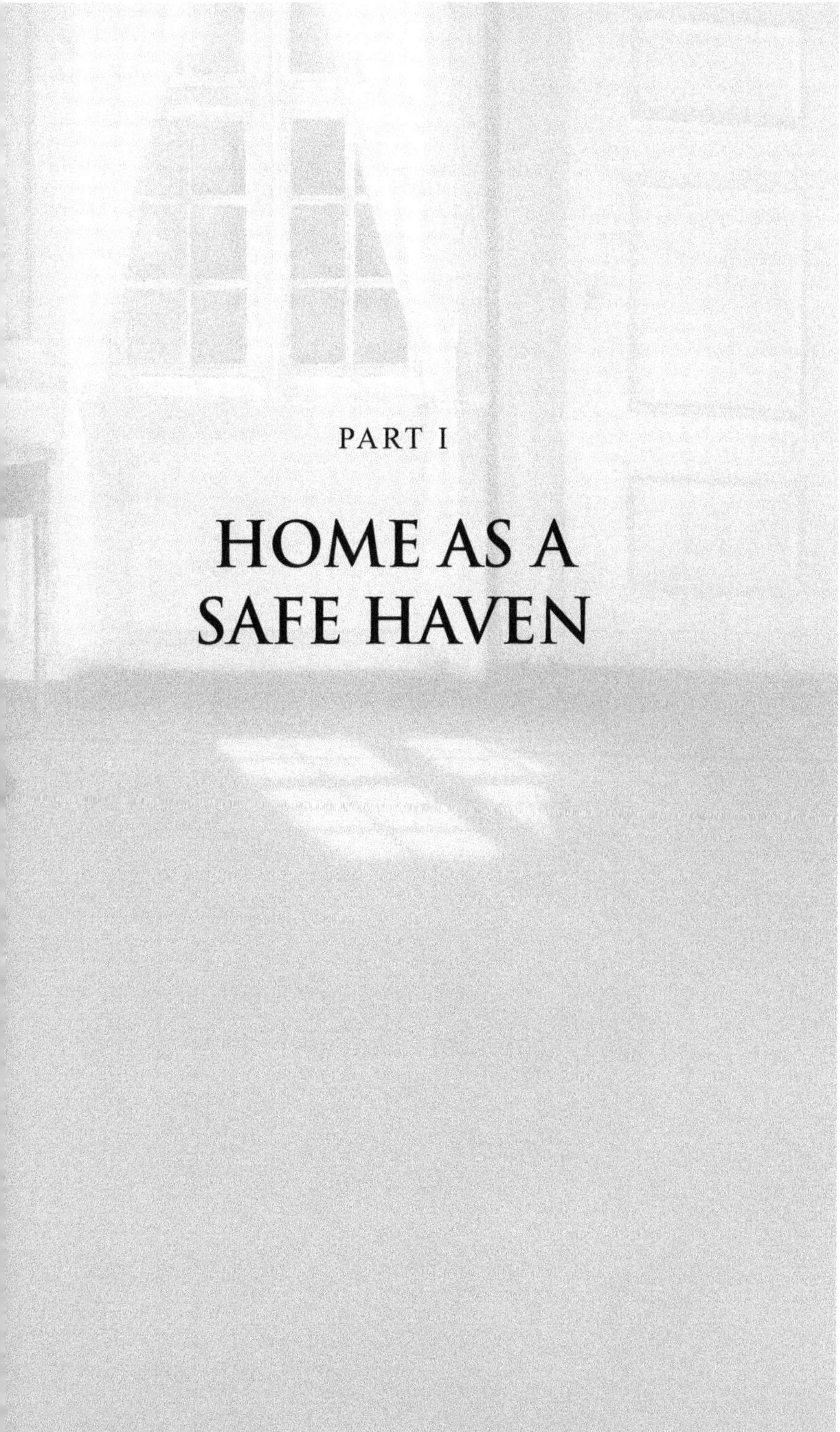

PART I

# HOME AS A
# SAFE HAVEN

# CHAPTER ONE

..................................................

# The Poetry of Place

## By Frank Beck

When Lou Andreas-Salomé met Sigmund Freud in 1910, she was better known than he. Her four novels and her studies of Ibsen and Nietzsche resonated powerfully with many German-speaking readers in the years before the First World War. Andreas-Salomé later studied with Freud and entered private practice as an analyst. Over time, she became his confidante, as well as a beloved friend and colleague of his daughter, Anna—their correspondence fills more than a thousand pages. After the war, she treated survivors with post-traumatic stress.

Raleigh Whitinger and I had long admired Andreas-Salomé's fiction, so we collaborated on a translation of her sixth and final novel (*Das Haus,* published in 1921), which we retitled *Anneliese's House.* Here a woman in her late thirties questions the choices she has made as a wife and mother, after giving up hopes of becoming a pianist. This is also the story of a hillside house that serves as an anchor for family life. Andreas-Salomé views it as the setting for love, anger, despair, and reconciliation—the high points in the unfolding of our relationships. As we worked on the book,

I found myself considering how home appears in Western literature and reviewing my own longing for this important place in our lives.

When poets and playwrights speak of home, it's often in passing. Rosalind declares "I wish I were at home" in Act IV of *As You Like It*, yet this is simply a sign that she's overcome, after hearing of her lover's battle with a lion, and that's the end of it. Even that inveterate homebody Hamlet has nothing to say on the subject. And what about modern writers? Dylan Thomas's "Poem on his birthday" is a rhapsodic tribute to the Welsh seaside town where he lived, but he only mentions the home he shared with his wife and three children as a "house on stilts high among beaks/and palavers of birds."

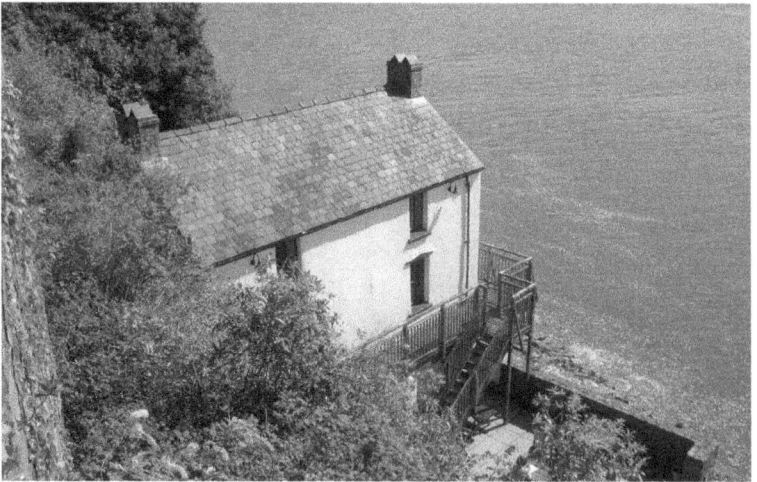

Dylan Thomas (1914-1953) lived and worked in his boathouse in Laugharne on Carmarthen Bay in Wales. Photo by Bryan Ledgard, Peter Broster, CC BY 2.0 <https://creativecommons.org/licenses/by/2.0>, via Wikimedia Commons

Why this absence of home? And why do some poets take this place for granted?

In many agrarian societies, a newly married couple would join the household of the husband's father, planning to inherit his fields, vines, and livestock, just as someone today inherits a bond portfolio. Home was not a place we, as individuals, invented, but something that lived on in us over time. Not just as a memory but as the stuff of life. Of course, the modern age has put an end to of that. Ever since the industrial revolution, we've been rolling stones. Now every generation loses touch with home in its own way.

Like many people who came of age in the 1960s, I spent my youth in a series of furnished rooms, rented houses, and apartments, never imagining any of these places would be my home for long. Still, I knew the kind of home I wanted. I was writing, and I believed writers needed the quiet of the country: I thought of Dylan Thomas, in his seaside home in Wales; Robert Frost, high in the mountains of New Hampshire; Boris Pasternak in his dacha outside Moscow. I indulged these bucolic fantasies while residing in New Brunswick, an easy commute to my job in Manhattan, in the steamship business, booking cargo that sailed to Bremen, Oslo and Helsinki—places I wished I were heading to for inspiration.

In those years, as I lived in different towns and traveled to many others in my imagination, I experienced the sense of rootlessness that Rainer Maria Rilke describes in his poem "Autumn Day" (*Herbsttag).* As a young man, Rilke left his native city of Prague and had eight addresses in Paris, interrupted by extended stays in Spain, Russia, Sweden, and Egypt. He didn't have a fixed abode until he was 45. He first went to Paris in September 1902 to write a monograph about Rodin, leaving his wife and daughter in Germany and staying in a student hotel near the Luxembourg Gardens. That's where he wrote so movingly about homesickness. Here's my translation:

> Lord, it is time. The summer was so great.
> Now lay your shadow across the sundials,
> And let the winds of the field run free.
>
> Tell the last of the grapes to ripen:
> give them two more days of southern warmth,
> urge them to completion, and then chase
> one final sweetness into the heavy vines.
>
> He who has no house now will not build one.
> He who is alone will be that way a long time.
> He'll lie awake and read and write long letters,
> and, up and down along the avenues,
> will wander anxiously, when brown leaves scatter.

In my youth, I longed to find someone who would help me find contentment in a single place. My first daughter was born in 1968, but my marriage ended soon afterward, and none of my other relationships lasted. I watched as my friends settled down. I sat on their lawns on summer evenings in the country, looking at the stars, and shared in their conversation, over late-night dinners in their city apartments. Yet I was only an observer of homes and happiness, like the creature in Thomas Hardy's "The Fallow Deer at the Lonely House."

> One without looks in tonight
>    Through the curtain chink
> From the sheet of glistening white;

One without looks in tonight
    As we sit and think
    By the fender-brink.

We do not discern those eyes
Watching in the snow;
Lit by lamps of rosy dyes
We do not discern those eyes
    Wondering, aglow
    Four-footed, tiptoe.

While I was working in that busy steamship office and trying to write in my spare time, I also discovered Robert Lowell's poem "The Old Flame"—a work that tantalized me with the pleasures of a happy home. Here Lowell revisits the house in Maine he had shared with his wife Elizabeth Hardwick. Years later, it sits empty: "Everything has been swept bare,/furnished, garnished and aired." But the poet offers up a wistful memory of the couple snowbound "in our tent of books."

Poor ghost, old love, speak
with your old voice
of flaming insight
that kept us awake all night.
In one bed and apart,

we heard the plow
groaning up hill—
a red light, then a blue,
as it tossed off the snow
to the side of the road.

This is what marriage must be, I thought. Listening to those simple sounds. Sharing the hush of the snow and the noises that keep us awake in the dark of night.

Just when I had nearly given up on that kind of companionship, I started dating a friend who was also a writer. She urged me to get out of the steamship business and get a job in publishing—and to keep working on my poems. We married, and soon had a daughter. Home, for all three of us, has long been a two-bedroom apartment in upper Manhattan, in Morningside Heights. And I've learned that writers can also thrive in cities, as Thomas Hardy did in London, Federico García Lorca in Granada, Ingeborg Bachmann in Rome.

A few weeks after I met my wife-to-be, I imagined a place where I could still hear echoes of my childhood but that would also have a soul and personality of its own.

> I remember these days when they come,
> sometime on the edge of summer
> and not so interested in its arduous work—
> wheat labors up under hot sun somewhere else.
>
> The whole sky's now the warm white of a sink.
> From a nearby window, the clink and clatter
> of dishes being dried and stacked out of sight.
> Each pot hung here's delighted with its place.
>
> Curtains rise gently as a sleeper's chest.
> The sweep of the clock's second hand is smoother.
> I saw an afternoon like this one first
> from eyes at the level of a cupboard door.

The same even light borne like a brimming glass.
As the spoon stirred, it made the pitcher ring
and filled the room with smells of lemonade.
My mother made our lives above me with her hands.

Noon's harsh bustle has receded like surf.
Things seen reach deeper in me, taking rest.
Each bone in my body had forgotten how it feels:
the ceaseless movement of unbroken calm.

Over the course of thirty years, my wife and I have made such
a nest. Looking around our apartment, I see something like
an archaeological record of our lives. The Post-Impressionist
paintings and the 18th-century furniture we inherited from
her family; the books we read and discussed, from Sophocles
to Alice Oswald; the music by Bach, Mozart, Schubert, and
Elgar we listened to; the handmade baskets and ceramics we
brought back from Europe, Mexico, and North Africa. Yet
both my wife and I still carry the imprint of our childhood
homes—and this kind of early memory continues to shape
each one of us to the end of life.

I was reminded of this last year, when I returned to
my parents' house to help care for my aging father. Hale and
hardy at 94, he had one problem: his mind was unraveling.
And last year, just before Christmas, his body failed, as well.
He was in and out of rehab facilities, and much of his last
three months he spent in a hospital bed in the living room.
My mother, my brother, and I made him as comfortable as we
could and settled in for the duration. Suddenly, I was back in a
pre-industrial, multi-generational household, with an ancient
rhythm to our daily lives. I thought of Odysseus who spent so

many years trying to get home not only to his wife and son, but to his father, Laertes, who was growing old.

One of the foundational poems of Western culture is the story of a man's struggle to return to his family home after an absence of twenty years. The Greeks prized these reunions. As Homer points out, the lesser deities may rule the sun, wind, and sea, but Zeus himself is the god of householders. On his return, Odysseus has difficulty persuading his father Laertes of his true identity. He displays a scar from a childhood injury, but Laertes remains unmoved. Yet when the two walk together in the orchard, Odysseus calls up the proper memory. Here is that scene from Book 24, in Emily Wilson's superb translation.[16]

> When I was little, I would follow you
> around the garden, asking all their names.
> We walked beneath these trees: you named them all
> and promised them to me. Ten apple trees,
> and thirteen pear trees, forty figs, and fifty
> grapevines, which ripen one by one—their clusters
> change as the weather presses from the sky,
> sent down by Zeus." At that Laertes' heart
> and legs gave way; he recognized the signs
> Odysseus had given as clear proof.
> He threw both arms around his ruthless son,
> who caught him as he fainted . . .

It was hard to see my own father too frail to walk more than a few steps, too weak to sit with us at the dining table. Yet, he still had one wish, and it astonished us. As he lay in bed in the house he'd shared with his wife since 1952, he insisted,

28

again and again, that he wanted to "go home." Where? To the small apartment along the train tracks in Elizabeth, New Jersey, where, in his confusion, he thought he might still find his mother.

In "Intimations of Immortality," Wordsworth refers to "thoughts that do often lie too deep for tears." If poetry speaks little about our love of home, perhaps it's because that love is too deep for words—and as instinctive as an infant grasping at a mother's breast. The feeling of our first home persists long after we have learned to thrive on our own. After a lifetime of trying one place after another, we still hope to reinvent that moment of primal and nearly perfect bliss.

*Frank Beck is a New York-based writer and translator who has critiqued new poetry for The Manhattan Review for more than 30 years. His latest thoughts on the arts can be found at DieHoren.com. With Raleigh Whitinger, he has published the first English translation of Lou Andreas-Salomé's novel* Anneliese's House, *a tale that draws on depth psychology to explore the joys and challenges of family life.*

# CHAPTER TWO

............................................................

## Typology at Home

### By Sally V. Keil

Personality tests like the Myers-Briggs are often given in the workplace to create ideal teams and foster collaboration. There's the manager known for quick thinking, the sensation type who designs inspiring presentations, the intuitive in charge of research and development, and the feeling type who keeps everyone engaged. Typology describes how we approach and understand our environment. How do we solve problems and relate to others? In a new situation, what is our gut instinct?

I first embarked upon my study of typology in my job in corporate marketing, where I drew on my intuition to make sense of the information I was gathering, and on my feeling function to navigate the department's emotional dynamics. As a result, there was always someone sitting in my office wanting counsel for some painful issue—work or personal— they were struggling with. Over the years, however, I got my best and most lasting insights by observing the personalities of my family members where they were most themselves—at home. This experience so enriched my life that I was inspired to write a book applying Jung's typology in daily life, *To Live in the World as Ourselves.*

I learned a good deal by noticing how the people I was closest to naturally did things, and how their orientation was different from mine. Couples are often drawn to one another because each has a different strength. At the beginning, they naturally complement each other. Then they have the task of learning to appreciate one another's way of being in the world. My husband Sean, an extravert, can't wait to leave the house in the morning, and as an introvert, I prefer the quiet solitude of my home office. At first, I thought, "How could he possibly want to charge forth like that, first thing?" But I've come to understand that he's wired, psychologically, to thrive when out and about, and I smile as he goes off on his adventures. I also appreciate Sean's need to share what he's discovered, and, at the end of every day, I look forward to his recap.

Typology also helped me in the years I was getting to know my three step-children, making it easy to spot and nurture their particular gifts. When I took my sensation-gifted daughter, Sara, with me to an art class, and to a gallery show, these shared experiences nourished our relationship. My other stepdaughter, Megan, is an intuitive like me, so we engaged in those sparky conversations full of "what-ifs" and "that-reminds-me," ranging from one topic to another, without following any logical progression. This way of relating I've come to call Intuitive's Delight. My stepson, Sean, who is sensation-endowed, noticed the least little change I made in the house, and it became a game for him to identify these alterations. Both introverts, we often met in the kitchen after everyone had gone to bed and talked quietly while sharing a beer. As I came to appreciate the natural inclinations of my stepchildren, genuine relationships were built.

In addition, typology also helped me understand my family of origin. My father's extreme introversion explained why conversations with him were few and far between, and why he disappeared after dinner to the focused calm of his workbench in the basement. My two sisters are also different from me typologically. One is an extraverted feeling type whose powerful feelings I found distressing until I realized that this was her natural way of processing events and venting helped her come to a resolution. My other sister, a thinking type and a natural born teacher, had a very smart, practical way of dealing with fourth graders. I gratefully drew on her skills in the course of creating a stepfamily.

"Typology in close quarters" might well be the subject of many psychotherapy sessions. Nothing spoils the feeling of home like conflict and misunderstanding. Yet, knowing everyone's natural typology can do wonders for our relationships and pave the way for domestic harmony. It is simply a case of recognizing what other people need to be fully and completely themselves.

As my understanding of typology grew, I left my corporate job and became a psychological counselor and freelance writer. As an introvert, I had discovered that I was happier working at home than I was managing the often-Machiavellian subtleties of office politics. While I learned a lot from my colleagues, I made beneficial changes after observing myself and recognizing my own patterns. Accepting my affinity for solitude, and my reliance on my intuition, has helped me to live more authentically. It has also brought a greater sense of confidence and self–esteem, allowing me to feel more at home within myself.

Everyone knows psychological awareness is desirable, but how do we go about attaining it? Knowing if you are introverted or extraverted, and if you naturally process information through thinking, feeling, sensation or intuition, is a good start. One that will allow you to begin living as yourself. And once you understand how the people around you are perceiving and processing the world, your relationships will make more sense. There's much to be said for meeting people where they are.

A harmonious home life for a busy family is a challenge. Creating the feeling of sanctuary involves knowing what you—and your loved ones—need your home to be. If you are extraverted, a friendly open common space where everyone can gather is essential. If you are introverted, you need to have a space where you can relax, regroup, write, read or do projects. My stepdaughter, Megan, an extravert, lives with two introverts, her husband and daughter. After dinner, they happily retreat to work or read, while Megan starts her evening with phone calls, texting and planning weekend activities. Later the family gathers in the living room for a tv show or movie, ending the day together.

Jung's insights are a boon to conscious parenting. A child thrives when his or her typology is honored. My stepson, Sean, the introvert, comes from a lively Irish tribe but I noticed he would stand at the periphery of family parties or duck out from time to time. His family worried that there was something wrong with him, but I suggested to him that he might be an introvert — he wasn't made to be the boisterous center of attention and he might prefer relating to people one-on-one. A lightbulb went off. From then on, when he'd had enough intense socializing, he would announce, "I'm an introvert!" and leave the room. Everyone would laugh, but they also acknowledged his preferences with real love and respect.

In typology, a little bit of our opposite mode goes a long way, because the experience is so powerful. When Sean grew up, he became an amazingly effective sales rep, but he knew to turn off his phone on Sundays and to ground himself by spending that day quietly at home.

For an introvert, home is exceptionally important. I have always needed home to be a quiet place where I can find solitude and where I can breathe, move, and think at my own pace. I currently live in a house big enough for a family of 11 plus the dog, but I relish times I get the house to myself. Alone time is vital for introverts to segue into to a busy family life. Others mustn't take it as a rejection; it is a psychological necessity. But to make that clear in a gentle way requires some effort. When I'm working in my office, my family knows to knock. They are always welcome, but there is no barging in. Virginia Woolf, a famous introvert, used to put a sign up on her door, "Writer at work" and another when she was in the mood for visitors that said in effect, "Come on in." Introverts are wise to provide these cues. For them, silence is a daily need.

Home is our best medium for understanding human behavior. There we are most likely to let down our guard and reveal ourselves. It's also one place where we hope to be natural. When we share our space with others, we also want it to reflect our personality—to embody who we really are. How do we accomplish that when we move in with others? I think back to the early days of my relationship with Sean. When we got engaged, I moved into his apartment, and we began to combine our lives and our possessions. Sean, who has a high-ranking sensation function, had already created an attractive and comfortable place to live. I loved his sensibility and didn't want to change it, but I did want to make my contribution, so I came up an enhancement that was not too radical: I hired a friend who was a feng shui master to evaluate the space. She suggested adding mirrors as splash boards behind the kitchen cooktop to accentuate the hearth, and also along the sides of the windows to bring in more light. These changes were beautiful and in keeping with the natural spirit of the home. She also placed some crystals in the hallway to disperse intergenerational conflict and suggested placing a plant in a certain corner of the living room. With those changes, the apartment was subtly transformed, and it felt like my space, too.

Sensation—the function that relies upon our physical perception—is key when it comes to creating a comfortable home. When you rely upon your sensation function, you are attuned to color, sound, and taste, especially aware of softness and roughness, warmth and coldness. The sensation function knows how to select the most sensuous sheets and how to appreciate a summer breeze wafting through an open window. We exercise our sensation when we shop for a cozy chair, select fabrics, arrange furniture, pick out vegetables at the market. And we call upon it to perform a myriad of housekeeping tasks—as we do the laundry, wipe our counter tops, wash dishes, make our beds, and care for our clothes.

Two sensation types I know live in a 750-square-foot apartment with their two children. This is a compact space for a family of four, but these sensation-gifted parents have designed a perfectly functional and beautiful family home. Every piece of furniture is the perfect size. Colors are serene, patterns harmonious, textures varied. Closets are packed but well-organized. And every cubic inch from floor to ceiling is well managed, so there is no sense of clutter. And this sense of "rightness" remains when a new thing is added, or the drapes are changed. This is what the sensation function does as a matter of course. In this world, small or big is beautiful.

But what if sensation activities don't interest you or tire you? How much of these activities can you do, and how much will you enjoy doing them? If sensation is a talent you rely upon, it will come easily. However, if you're an intuitive like me, it may be a challenge. I need to know that everything is in its place, or my environment feels overwhelming. Many intuitives choose to keep their homes stable and unchanging. One intuitive friend hasn't moved so much as a chair in 15 years. She has created a set environment that works for her, allowing her to concentrate on her writing and her inner world.

Jung developed his system of typology from his own experience—from observing himself, his family members, his colleagues and his patients, and learning how they behaved at home. Typology is built into human nature and is the ultimate inner journey. It's both a form of hard-wiring and a form of revelation. The more aware we are of the typological aspects of any situation, the more at ease we feel.

Home is the source of intimacy and relationships, the place where we learn how to develop empathy, self-awareness and respect for one another's uniqueness. It's where we pay attention to our needs and learn to navigate the needs of others. And it's the laboratory where we grow in understanding and begin to live as our true selves.

*Sally V. Keil is a psychological counselor who also writes about mythology, dreams, and women's lives. Her latest book is* To Live in the World as Ourselves: Self-Discovery and Better Relationships through Jung's Typology.

# CHAPTER THREE

...................................................

# The Mythology of the Man Cave

## By Anthony Lawlor

The poet Gary Snyder observes, "All of us carry within us caves; with animals and gods on the walls; a place of ritual and magic." Long before men retreated to suburban basements lugging flatscreen TV's, overstuffed recliners, chips, and beer, they descended into subterranean caves carrying ritual masks, paint kits, drums and flutes. On the surface, the comfortable escapes inhabited by 21st century men seem worlds apart from the dark, stony initiation chambers fashioned by their ancient brothers. The carpeted contemporary cave and the jagged cleft in the earth, however, share common foundations in the male psyche.

I recall my first encounter with a prototypical male cavern in a remote area of New Mexico. On a scorching August afternoon, I strode across the parched earth towards a log ladder poking skyward from the ground. The glare of the sun was so intense, I had to shield my eyes. A torrid breeze did little to help, as beads of sweat rolled from the back of my neck down my spine. In the surrounding trees, I heard the constant drone of insects. When I reached the ladder, I grasped the side rails and lowered myself rung by rung through a 24-inch square opening until I found firm purchase on the clay floor of the kiva.

This interior space was the yin to the upper world's yang. Harsh sunlight, baking temperature, a hot wind and roaring insects had given way to darkness, cool stillness and silence. The chamber's circular shape gave the impression of an edgeless spaciousness. Soon my breathing slowed, my shoulders relaxed, and my mind eased into restful awareness. Every part of me felt welcomed by this place. I was home.

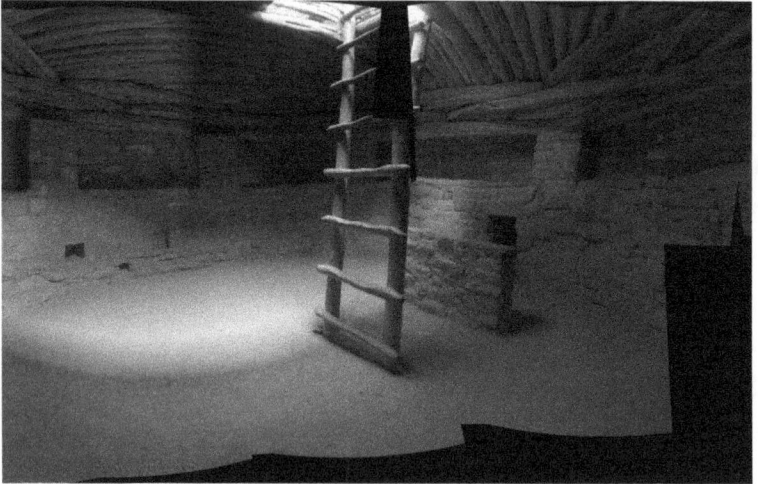

Kiva in New Mexico, *CC BY-SA 3.0,*
*https://commons.wikimedia.org/w/index.php?curid=1103129*

In the murky light, I made my way to the earthen bench that ran along the curved wall of the kiva. Settling into the darkness, the shaft of sunlight flooding through the square opening was decidedly masculine, like a sword piercing the space—while the kiva was like an architectural womb. In Jung's theory of the collective unconscious, the feminine side of a man needs to come into greater awareness, and many of our current problems today stem from men being out of touch with their feelings and this feminine aspect of themselves. This kiva provided a womb-like setting for me to engage my relationship to the feminine, which Jung called the anima. I hadn't come here with the intention of having such an encounter, but this subterranean cavern had a profound effect—one that was impossible to ignore.

Dropping into the silence of the kiva, I sensed the forces of birth and death, order and chaos, conscious and unconscious, meaning and absurdity, reason and imagination and other opposing forces stirring within my psyche. The kiva called me to go beyond the describable limits of thinking, into ineffable depths of being. This experience was at once simple and profound, settling and unsettling, strange and familiar. My senses were fully alive. The muffled whoosh of my breathing and the quiet scrape of my fingertips on the clay bench resonated in this enclosed space like temple bells. The feeling of the adobe wall against my back felt strong, stable, comforting. I was serene and radiantly awake.

In my explorations of world architecture, I am consistently drawn to cave-like spaces. Our Lady of Chartres, the magnificent Gothic cathedral outside of Paris, has a dark, cavernous interior where stained glass windows glow like jewels displayed on black velvet. The church is an elaborately constructed womb where I have had clear and powerful encounters with the feminine. Inside the western entry doors of the cathedral is the famous labyrinth, embossed in the limestone floor. Treading its twisting, turning path I am reminded that life does not always proceed logically and rationality, nor does history unfold in a straight line. Here I sense the earthy, fluid, receptive and intuitive forces at work in the unconscious, and at work in the world. The parallel to the piercing masculine in the kiva is the enormous rose window that seems afire on the west wall of the cathedral. The labyrinth and the rose window are juxtaposed in an architectural marriage of masculine and feminine forces.

When these opposites aren't acknowledged, a place lacks meaning and vitality, as in the contemporary cathedral of Évry, near Paris. Inside the building, I found a circular space flooded with brightness from the skylight covering most of the ceiling. This church was so overly illumined that it felt like a cafeteria. There was no depth or mystery. I longed for the dim lighting and glowing stained glass of Chartres Cathedral that provides layers of shadow, containing the elusive secrets of creation.

What happens when we apply this mythology to the modern man cave? The flat screen television is the major focal point of the typical basement escape. It is here we watch our masculine rituals of triumph and defeat and see our heroes on the playing field overcome great obstacles in dazzling color. This is a scene that would be familiar to the Greeks, who also knew a thing or two about framing.

On a bright November morning, I climbed the hill north of the harbor on the island of Naxos. My eye was immediately drawn to a rectangle of white marble standing amidst the ancient ruins of a temple dedicated to Apollo. Moving closer, I felt dwarfed by this 20-foot tall, 12-foot-wide white stone frame. Standing in this colossal gateway, I looked up at a patch of dazzling blue Mediterranean sky. Within this geometric space, I saw what I can only describe as energy, trembling without moving, rumbling without making a sound. The moment was charged, potent like the instant before striking a match in a dark room or before the first stroke of the violin pierces the silence of a concert hall. This marble frame pointed my awareness beyond itself to something larger and more mysterious, and I suddenly understood that great architecture, design and art call us to go beyond a physical space and enter a transcendent realm.

Cinematographers rely upon the power of the frame to convey a change of character or fate. In *The Shawshank Redemption*, Andy has been planning his escape from prison for years; he has dug a tunnel from the wall of his cell into a sewage pipe, and finally crawls to freedom through 500 yards of shit-smelling filth. As he emerges from this underworld, he tears off his prison shirt and raises his arms skyward toward the pouring rain. For a moment, he is standing in that frame that promises new life and liberation.

Men have such experiences in their creative lives today, whether they are writers, artists, scientists, entrepreneurs or craftsmen.

Men need a place to escape the world of daily responsibility. This is in our DNA—this need for an archetypal passage to the underworld, for an initiation into caverns and dark womb-like spaces. We need dens where we can confront our fears, where our innermost powers can be strengthened and renewed. Formalized versions of masculine caves, men's clubs in New York and London, sought to replicate this too, with their rules against talking or doing any business on the premises. Men aren't allowed to bring their briefcases into the bar or library. They must be checked. This is for good reason! We need to have a least one portion of our lives that isn't dictated by the God of Economics.

I recall Virginia Woolf's advice that each woman needs "a room of her own" in order to discover her own creativity. For centuries, men have relied on that tradition. Sometimes that room is a library where books become sacred portals; an atelier, where they draw or paint; or a workbench, where they make something beautiful and useful.

As an architect with great concern for "interiors," I encourage men to establish a place where they can encounter the Muse and explore the depths of their creativity.

My own private space revolves around my writing and drawing desk. Beside my computer, I have placed a small brass Tibetan bowl-shaped bell, a wood Native American flute, and some brushes and paints. On the wall are photographs I've taken during my travels to sacred architectural sites, and some of my own sketches. Here I leave behind daily concerns and dive deep into the cave of my imagination. Like the kiva, my room is a dark and womb-like place. Like the Rose Window at Chartres it reminds me of that "aha" moment of illumination. And like the ruins at the Greek temple of Apollo, it provides a portal to another world.

*Anthony Lawlor is an award-winning architect and author of* The Temple in the House *and* A Home for the Soul. *His work has been featured on National Public Radio, The Oprah Winfrey Show and numerous other media outlets. He is currently exploring the possibilities of sanctuary at his cottage in northern California.*

# CHAPTER FOUR

## Renovating with a Shaman

### By Gilda Frantz

My personal experiences with shamanism began years ago. My husband's younger sister was killed in a plane crash, and we stored all of her belongings. My mother-in-law died of old age in the early 1960s, so we took her belongings and stored them in our garage. My older sister passed away in 1968, and because her children were young and not settled in their lives, I agreed to store some of her belongings until they grew up—into our garage they went. Then my brother-in-law died suddenly, and his children also were living in places without much storage, so they stored some and we stored some. In 1975 my husband died suddenly and left an entire medical library as well as records of patients. Into the garage they went to be stored.

My son died in 1992 and I had all his things to store. So went my life, divided between the profound losses and having to deal with "things" left behind.

Then, one day about ten years ago, I decided to create a guesthouse out of the garage. My thinking was that since I couldn't access the garage for my car, I might as well use it to host visiting friends. I had plans drawn up for a cozy bedroom, living room, kitchen, and bath. It was going to be a darling little house nestled in my garden. I would keep the shell and change the interior.

There was only one major problem: I found it impossible to go into this garage to begin the clearing-out process, as it was damp, moldy, and sad. I used to say it was like a mausoleum where the dead were stored. I didn't believe the spirits of my beloved relatives and husband were there, but the smell of books that had become moldy in the damp beach climate was pervasive—and unpleasant. I would open the door to enter and turn around and leave.

I knew I had to do something, so I did what I do at such times: I called my daughter and asked her what she would do in a similar situation.

She immediately suggested that I call Miguel. I wondered how Miguel might help, but I trust her intuition and called him at once. Miguel married my late husband's great-niece Stephanie. Born and raised in Guatemala, Miguel has a shock of longish white hair and a very soft voice. He was called to study with Native Americans and considers one Native American healer, in particular, as his teacher. Miguel leads sweat lodge ceremonies and supervises vision quests on a regular basis. My daughter has participated in these rituals and has high regard for Miguel.

I arranged with him to come to my house, and he arrived with an arm-load of things. I took him to the garage. I sat with my little Pug, Mr. Fu, on my lap, and Miguel began a ceremony to help me let go of these possessions. First, he filled a small container with herbs and lit it, releasing a sweet and pungent fragrance in the smoke wafting in the air.

I drifted into a kind of reverie, although I was aware of his opening a beautiful lined carrying case in which he stored two hawk wings, which he held aloft while chanting and drumming. I began to breathe slowly as a deep ease spread throughout me.

After quite a while, maybe an hour or more, Miguel stopped chanting and turned to the walls where the artifacts were stored on shelves. In effect, he asked the objects to "Let go of Gilda." It was stunning to hear him choose those words, as it had never occurred to me that these objects were holding on to me, even though I remembered that Jung felt his kitchen tools "acted up" when he left them for a long time and he would apologize to them upon his return. Miguel, in his gentle voice, implored the objects to understand that they would go on to another life if they gave Gilda a chance to grow, too.

Then it was over. Miguel packed his things carefully and respectfully and we said goodbye. I later learned that what he was chanting that I couldn't understand were prayers in a Native American language.

The next morning, I went to the door of the garage, opened it, and entered.

The moldy odor had evaporated, and I didn't feel weird or sad entering this sacred space. Eventually I gave things away and, in some instances, had to toss objects that were too far-gone with mold. I did it with respect and love for the previous owner. My friend Miguel had changed the very energy in the garage, and I could enter and do what was necessary.

*Gilda Frantz, M.A, was a senior Jungian analyst in Santa Monica specializing in creativity and loss. This piece originally appeared in Psychological Perspectives, 57: 123– 125, 2014 as "Shamanic and Magical Realms." Copyright, C. G. Jung Institute of Los Angeles.*

# CHAPTER FIVE

## Far from the Irish Sea

### By John Hill

Home structures the story of our lives. Mine began in Ireland in a cloud of unknowing. I was told that I cried so much in the first few months of my life that I had to be operated on for a ruptured hernia.

In my 4th year, I contracted tuberculosis, discovered accidentally while I was staying with relatives in England. Unable to walk, I created an imaginary home inhabited by imaginary parents during the two years I was in the hospital. I believe those imaginary homescapes and the regular visits by a faithful aunt helped me survive an ordeal that my mind could barely acknowledge.

Eventually I learned to walk again and returned to Ireland. I remained fragile and was sent to a boarding school with only five pupils run by a German Baron and his wife. They were forced by the Nazis to leave their homeland and created in Ireland a school inspired by Rudolf Steiner by whom they had been befriended. It became my second home. I remember the affection and tenderness of that old couple who taught me to appreciate the beauty of nature. Still, today, I remember the dark woods, winding rivers, and sparkling lakes, all alive with wondrous creatures. My attachment to the earth was further strengthened through our lessons on nature, often held under an old willow tree.

Having grown up on the edge of the Irish Sea, I was familiar with the ocean that continually changes and mirrors the mysterious origins of human nature. Its violent storms and reassuring tidal rhythms, its myriad shapes and colors, celebrate life's intensity and diversity. For months I would sit on the seashore and talk with the ocean: "Sea, you touch every land on the planet, you hold the secrets of my life. Show me your ways."

As a young man, I walked the docks, approaching new ships for work, hoping the sea would take me to the next station of my life. I was lucky that some of those ships did not invite me onboard, otherwise I probably would not be alive to tell this tale. Finally, an old cargo ship on its last voyage accepted me as a member of the Royal Merchant Navy of Norway, starting as a cabin boy cleaning toilets. After an odyssey of five months through many lands, I found myself studying to become a psychoanalyst at the Jung Institute in Zurich.

When I arrived in Switzerland, home became marriage, children and profession. Despite financial stress in the first 10 years of family life, I don't think I ever felt more secure and fulfilled than I did in sharing a home with a loving and loyal wife, partaking in the life and development of two wonderful boys. My family life was definitely matrilocal. My social life extended only to my wife's family and friends. Later we lived in a beautiful wooden house in Einsieldn, a small town with a massive basilica that houses the Black Madonna and is situated near a picturesque lake nestled in the majestic Alpine landscape. For many hours I worked the soil, transforming the rather plain Swiss garden into a landscape of rocks and boulders, embellished with colorful shrubs and flowers—little Ireland!

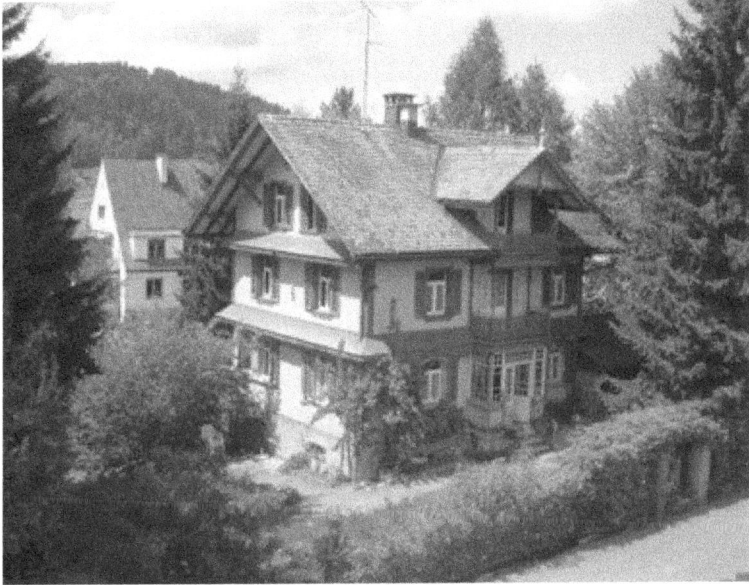

*The author's home in Einsiedeln. Courtesy of John Hill.*

There were, however, times when I became homesick for my native land and culture. Each year I revisited Ireland to reassure myself that my homeland would not disappear but survive as part of my identity. Dreams of Ireland's Celtic myths and modern Irish literature sustained my new life in Switzerland. As if to keep alive the memory of my original homeland, sensory images would return again and again—the sound of the sea, the smell of the turf, the lilt of Irish folk music.

Today, when I am away from Switzerland, I not only miss the music of the alphorn or the taste of Swiss pralines, but also the picturesque villages, the dark woods, and the majestic mountains of my adopted country. I must see, hear, or smell my home even when I am not physically in it—for as the French philosopher Merleau-Ponty said, the body is not an object among objects but our way of belonging to the world.

I assume most of us do not want to give up a secure life. I was no exception. I would have liked the gifts I received in the first half of life to last forever, but a midlife crisis with all its ambiguities and uncertainties ravished me. Women were telling me a tale I could not understand—some part of myself was not alive and they knew it. I eventually broke the home I had built and chose a solitary life, connected with a mature and free woman who lived in a land far away. This relationship was not about householding; its focus was on the recognition of a soul that animates body, heart, and mind, and has a different agenda than the conscious self. The pain of separation from the old and the comings and goings of the new forced me to develop a fierce independence.

I am grateful for all that happened during those years, yet my heart remains sorrowful for the pain I inflicted on people whom I have loved. I have learned to accept responsibility for who I am, for my strengths and weaknesses, to recognize the effects of traumatized stillborn parts of myself, and to care for them, preventing them from hurting the lives of others.

After having experienced the trials of midlife, I am now entering the final stage of life. I feel more rooted and at home in myself than ever before. I can accept the house that I have built, with its shine and its shadows. I have been able to translate, at least partially, the landscapes of Ireland into other homelands, particularly my adopted homeland

Switzerland and the Greek Isle of Patmos to which I return every year. My Irish soul delights in the sea, the barren rocks, and the little chapels of that holy island. I now have many loved ones—including my former wife, my children, dear friends, and professional colleagues with whom I have shared the drama of life.

Home has become a function of consciousness, a consensual concept, and a way of constructing relationships to those near and far, to the city and to the cosmos. Home is a work of art that takes a lifetime to create. Part of its story is contained in attachment to houses, gardens, animals, landscapes, schools, churches, ideas, music and works of art.

Home can also be understood as attachment to major attitudes that change during the course of one's life. The theologian Jürgen Moltmann once described the powerful forces that mold us: trust, in childhood; longing in youth; responsibility in maturity; and wisdom in old age.

I have always been impressed by the Indian notion that a woman is never without a husband. My heart seems to be saying that I have had four marriages: to mother, wife, soul, and death. I have felt at home in these marriages. The final one is still in the process of being built: it began soon after I reached midlife. It is the work of the spirit—a summing up and acceptance of one's life narrative, for better or for worse, in order to face the final challenge.

I hope that the shelters I have built for myself can, in different ways, provide shelter for others. I expect to take those shelters with me as I face the final question: Do we have a home that outlasts our short life on earth? Most of us will end our life on a mattress. That will be our final space on earth. I imagine the mattress could become a magic carpet that will carry me into unknown territory.

Schopenhauer examined the fabric of that last space we call home: "Life may be compared to a piece of embroidery, of which during the first half of his time, a man gets a sight of the right side, and during the second half, of the wrong. The wrong side is not so pretty as the right, but it is more instructive: It shows the way in which the threads have been worked together."

*This essay has been adapted from John Hill's book,* At Home in the World, *Chiron Publications, 2022. Hill is a psychoanalyst at the C.G. Jung Institute in Zurich. He has lived in Ireland, England, America, Switzerland, and Greece, and on a Norwegian merchant ship.*

# PART II

# HOME IN TIMES
# OF TRAUMA

# CHAPTER SIX

......................................................

## American Icarus

### By Pythia Peay

*American Icarus: A Memoir of Father and Country* follows my larger-than-life father, Joe, from his Dickensian childhood during the Depression to his years with the Air Transport Command in Brazil during World War II, then as a farmer in the Missouri heartland raising four children and working as a pilot for TWA. This is a searching portrait of a man who was never at home in his own skin, or with the sheer ordinariness of daily life. His story illuminates our American fascination with heroes and high-flyers, and their inevitable crashes.

Joe Carroll stood six-foot one inch tall, with blue eyes that could impale a person at a glance and a washboard stomach as hard as a balled fist. Zeus-like, he reigned over my childhood. Master of the stare-down, he could fix you motionless without a word. Once my brother Steven refused my father's order to get on the tractor and mow the alfalfa field; mouthing off with a smartass, "Fuck you." No one ever crossed my father, much less swore at him, and he backhanded my brother across his face hard, breaking his nose.

My father wasn't born a tyrant. In his youth he was beautiful, with a round and vulnerable face framed by neatly combed wavy brown hair. He had a deep dimple in his chin, full lips and wide eyes as bright as a pair of newborn stars. In one photo from the family album, he is a cocky, dapper lad leaning his elbow on a tree trunk beside his brothers and uncle. In another, he is a commanding young aviator standing on the runway with his flying buddies as they prepare to board a Douglas DC-4.

In yet others, he is a fresh-faced young husband coming to his wedding cake with his curly-haired bride standing next to him. Or a new father with his arms wrapped protectively around the chubby baby: me. Like a 1950s *Life* magazine ad, Joe Carroll's sparkling intensity leaps from these pictures radiating the hunger for life, raw optimism and an against-all-the-odds courage of an America that emerged from the depression to win World War II. The very air around him seems to vibrate with the bravado of a country about to enter the jet age of which he would be a part as a flight engineer for TWA.

What made Joe's moods hardest to figure out was that they did not emerge full-blown at the onset of our family life. No, they unspooled over the years like a mountain climber's rope staked to rock that unwinds slowly until, loosened, it snakes wildly out of control, dropping the person over the edge. Aimed straight at constructing a new life out of a childhood misshapen by the shock of loss and strange fortune, my father was at his strongest in the early years of our family. And so it was that my first memory of him as a little girl is that of tender love and exuberance for life and all its warm-earth sun-drenched beauty.

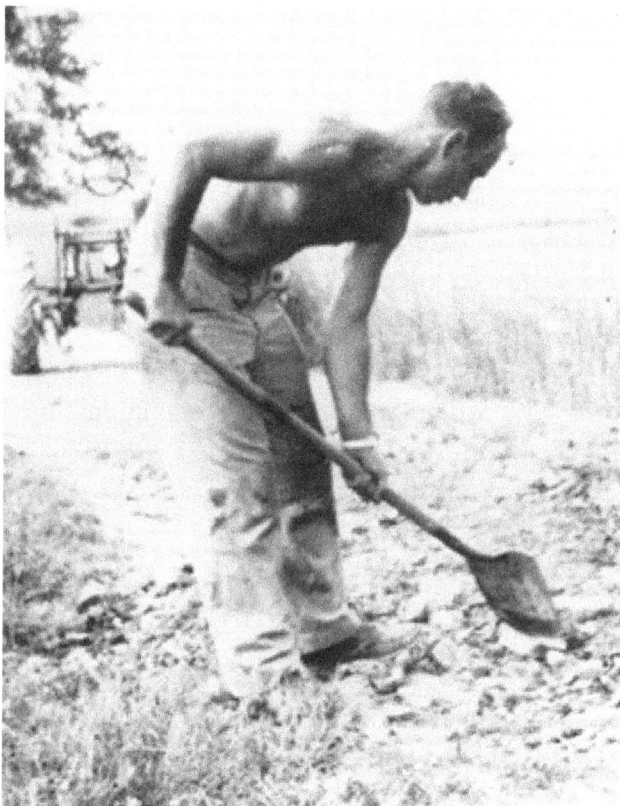

*Joe Carroll working on his farm, Shalom Acres.*

The very best days were the ones when Joe was getting ready to leave on a trip, or immediately after his return. Then there was a reassuring measure of order. There would be no scenes. The bottles of beer and vodka vanished, and the house bathed under the clean clear skies of sobriety. Preparing to leave, Joe whistled, shaved and packed. "Sheila!" he would call out to my mother, looking for the clean socks and pressed handkerchiefs he needed for his suitcase. Long into adulthood, I remember the lime aroma of Cannon aftershave and the crisp chemical smell of his newly dry-cleaned TWA uniform.

On a bad drinking day, it didn't take him long to get started. First came the Catholic grace over six bowed heads. "Thank you, Father, for that which we are about to receive," we would pray in unison, paying homage to the big daddy in the sky as well as at the table, and then it would begin.

"Stupid Lazy Hostesses!" he might say referring to the crew on his last flight, his eyes darting around the table. "Old Fat Cows!" he would mumble, glancing in my mother's direction hoping to draw someone into a showdown at the Carroll corral, then "Sheila! Lazy pig, where's the goddamn garlic bread?" he would bark, sending my mother flying from the room in a gush of tears. Mostly I sat hunched and mute before this gale force of paternal fury. Other times I took the bait, hurrying to the defense of my mother or the brother or sister or who had refused his I dare-you-to-disobey-me order to eat every last morsel of food on the plate.

The trickiest times of all, however, were when the good days collided with the bad, and my father became a dangerous brew of high spirits and brooding melancholy. When these high- and low-pressure systems came together my father was at his most charismatic: a pure force of human nature that combined everything terrible and wonderful at once. At moments like these, his starlit eyes flashed a rare brilliance that irradiated everyone around him with waves of energy.

One Sunday after mass when I was about 11, Joe theatrically unveiled his latest purchase: a new kind of electric sandwich maker that had long handles and a round press that neatly chopped off the edges of the bread, creating a perfectly spherical hot sandwich. With great flourish and fanfare, holding the press over the gas flame like a conductor waving his baton, dad cooked up his version of the Reuben sandwich. As a rule, I hated the bitter taste of sauerkraut, but something about Joe's juicy good humor made me love his corned beef and rye concoction, dripping with grainy mustard and melted Swiss cheese. My sister detested the hypocrisy of the Sunday morning brunches and wondered skeptically why Joe was suddenly trying to play the good father. But I loved them, carried aloft by my father's beguiling brand of wizardry that could turn a mere sandwich into food that I thought was fit for immortals.

There was nothing remotely mild or pallid about Joe. He met life full on, with everything he had. He could grind a field mouse beneath his heel, flail the horses with his long whip, and pick up the cat by its tail and hurl it across the field, causing me to squeal in fright and disgust. Or he could tenderly help my sister care for a litter of abandoned kittens, whistle an Irish ballad, or tell me a bedtime story with such pathos my eyes would fill with tears. He could, in equal measure, be boyish and happy or bullying and morose, generous and goodhearted or bitter and stingy, charming and loving or vindictive and hateful. He was a mess of contradictions and impossible to figure out.

As the years passed, the original masterpiece that was Joe's face became encrusted with the thick pigment of paranoia and despair. The more he drank the more I struggled to comprehend this increasingly difficult man Fate had chosen as my father. As a teenager, while a little unhinged from the uncertainty of it all, I would yell, cajole, and act out to get

Dad's attention, doing everything possible I could think of to save him.

When none of my schemes worked, and my own sanity seemed at risk, I knew it was time for me to get a life of my own. So I left—angrily and impetuously—willfully intent, if not on rescuing my father, then on saving the world instead. Swept up in the swelling counterculture movement, I glimpsed an opening to a new destiny. Driving from Missouri to California, I moved into a commune, found a spiritual teacher, and god.

When Icarus first soared upward, he only had eyes for the sun. But since then, the French launched the first man in hot air balloon. In 1783, flying had transfigured how we see Earth. During that first flight, one of the two pilots onboard became so distracted by the expansive view below him that he momentarily forgot his duties. As he stood up in the middle of the gondola, he found himself lost "in this spectacle offered by the immensity of the horizon. When I took off from the fields, the sun had set for the inhabitants of the valleys. Soon it rose for me alone."

But as much as flight would reveal Earth as a geographical wonder, a stupendous mystery, it would also show something else: its slow destruction. From space could be seen deforestation, oil spills, smog and urban sprawl.

When I reflect on the question my father pondered in the last days of his life—whether he was a flyer or a farmer—I wonder if I missed the larger point. In my mind, the real question that should've been asked was how flying shaped Joe's psychology, as well as his relationship to the land itself. Did flight inflate his dangerous tendency toward mania, urging him to take on more than his inborn limits would allow? Did it weaken his connection to the farm itself, causing the fields, barns, animals, and his wife and children to shrink in proportion to his life in the sky?

When I was around 15, an aerial photographer stopped by the house and proposed shooting a picture of the property from the sky. Joe loved this notion. At dinner that night, he spoke with animation about seeing the finished results. When we received the black-and-white photo, and after all of us had oohed and aahed over it, I proudly pasted it into a family album, with a hand-written caption, "The Carroll Family Farm."

Even before flight, America had from its beginnings had trouble being rooted in the land. Of Joe's twin loves, I realized it was flying that had come easiest to him; walking on the ground of his own life had proved the more difficult art. Ultimately, the farm would turn against him, and he too, would turn against the farm. I can't really blame my father for how things turned out. Besides, by living out the American dream of progress as fast and as hard as he could, he'd thought he was doing the right thing.

I keep on my writing desk two mementos from my father; his TWA wings and his tie clip, embellished with an image of a rocket lift off. Emblems of his career, they call me, still, to the rim of the weightless horizon. Just as Daedalus fit his son with the wings and feathers, and taught him the rules of flight, so my father imprinted on me the patterns of his life-myth. As my father had been smitten with sky-daring heroes like Charles Lindbergh and Howard Hughes, so too, had I gravitated to the edge of my time. Joining up with the raucous revolution of the 60s had been my way of following in my father's footsteps—even as I fled from home and tried to sever myself from his values. Where change was, where risk and excitement was, there I'd be. Sure enough, just as my father eventually crashed, so I also flew too near the blazing sun and fell back to Earth, a newly mortal teenager in a lonely hospital bed far from home.

The story of Icarus still speaks to us across the centuries because we recognize the familiar parable of flying high then falling low, rising to success and sinking to the nadir of failure; working hard and crashing; we're either flying high or being stone cold sober. The Greeks recognized this stance of extremes as the endless up and down of life.

The urge to touch the sun, to be greater than we are, is an especially exaggerated American trait. It is celebrated in every technological breakthrough, presidential inaugural speech, or American Idol contest. It is our spectacular, defining genius.

But it is also our tragic flaw. Through its lens, our history comes into focus. It is the Founding Fathers enshrining the principle of individual liberty in the Declaration of Independence. It is the genocide of the Native Americans and the sin of African American slavery. It is astronaut Neil Armstrong taking humankind's first step on the moon; it is the Challenger exploding into space. It is New York City's twin towers rising to touch the sky; it is terrorists in jets reducing them to rubble. It is a capitalist free-market that turns a poor cab driver into a wealthy entrepreneur—and then melts away his savings in an economic turndown, putting him back on the streets as a cabdriver once again.

And it is my father, sailing through the air in a jet only to return home to sit through the night drinking and grieving in darkness over the daughter who fled his house. As I learned from my father's life, we could begin to balance our culture of striving with a culture of healing and deepening, reconciling our compulsive drive for change with cultivating what we already have—in honor of that vast land we claim to love.

To do this, however, would mean overcoming our distrust of the inner life and embracing self-examination and even suffering, old-fashioned and anti-American as this may sound.

Writing this book about my father's life was a years-long journey of discovery, with many unexpected twists and turns—almost like a *Raiders of the Lost Ark* experience in the sense of recovering something precious—even holy. As a child, I had dreamt of being an archaeologist; as a journalist, how a nation is psychologically shaped by its past became my primary focus. When I began to research and write about my father, not long after he died, all these interests converged.

Drawing on conversations Joe had with his Hospice nurse about his childhood growing up during the Depression, I began to retrace the story of my father's life. From the time I got into my car to drive to Joe Carroll's birthplace in Altoona, Pa., to conversations with cousins I'd never met, interviews with military and aviation historians about his career as an aviator during the war, I realized there was much I didn't know about the man who'd raised me. Had my father been involved in undercover work for the FBI during World War II, as more than one aviation historian had alluded? Though told that this could never be officially "confirmed or denied," the very notion significantly shifted my idea of who my father was, and the secret life (or lives) he'd lived. Where before I had judged him for his silent withdrawals, erratic moods, and especially his drinking, I came to understand the link between his addiction and the PTSD endured by veterans of war, and the horrors they have seen, but cannot talk about.

Learning these things made me feel deeply sad that I hadn't been more sensitive to the conflicts Joe had wrestled with while he was alive. "Was I a farmer, or a flier?" he asked me during one particularly long and restless night, near the end of his life. "I'd really like to know."

Researching this book, I understood my father's conflict was not his alone, but reflected a larger American struggle between the heights of outward success and achievement, and the depths of feeling associated with family and nature. As I wrote, I found myself drawing closer to my father, and, as he came to me in dream after dream, he drew closer to me as well.

*Pythia Peay is known for her writing about psychology, spirituality, and the American psyche. Her work has appeared in The Washington Post, The Huffington Post and Psychology Today, and she is the author of* America on the Couch: Psychological Perspectives on American Politics and Culture. *She makes her home in Washington, D.C.*

## CHAPTER SEVEN

........................................................

# These Wilds Beyond Our Fences— Letters to My Daughter on Humanity's Search for Home

### By Bayo Akomolafe

I don't become your father the first time I hear you rip the air with your song or when I later carry you close to my chest, shaky and afraid that I might do something silly and drop you. I tend to think it is the moment we bring you to your grandmother's home, the house your maternal grandfather—a Nigerian like me—bought for his Indian wife. I steal away from the festivity of laughter often punctuated by *shhh! Lower-your-voice-she-still-is-sleeping* persuasions—and find a private spot. There, where no one else can hear, I say a short prayer to you. I make a promise to give you a home, to work for your future, to love you with my darkness, to be the ground upon which you stand, to create a whole new world. I promise to be your father.

I met a wild man once. He lives at the edges, where the wild things press their faces against the borders and make furry noises. He is a bank of many sorrows. Many griefs. He knows how to wheedle a hush—one of those creatures that crawl across the earth's meandering planes, and hide in the shadows of her belly folds—and speaks in incantations. He speaks in incantations and says a hush is not a trifling matter, that a hush has a message to share. To sit with a hush is to meet oneself as if for the first time. It is to come home. And *this,* coming home, is why I write you.

They say that when you're about to die your life flashes before you, you see those you love, those moments you cherish, in spontaneous psychic edits of final warning. Perhaps that is only true in specific situations where one is distant from loved ones. I need no private cinematic bursts of my life and my loved ones. I can see them already and they are about to be murdered by the gun of a Zairian child soldier who stands at the doorway watching us.

I don't know how long I've shut my eyes or how long this silence took me, but I can hear a conversation in Lingala. My ears seem to clear open, much in the same way stuffy ears are unclogged after one alights from a plane. Uncle Bernard is here and he seems to be translating the soldier's comments to my mum and dad. Uncle Bernard tells them that the soldier boy pities us. He saw my mother pray and since he is Christian, too, he will not take our lives, but that he doesn't know what his boss will do to him and that they will all be going soon—when they have taken all they want from our home.

So long as I live I will never forget the wave of relief that washes over my mother's splintered face as she collapses to the ground saying, "Thank you. Thank you. Ah, thank you!" I cannot see my father's face, just his back, but he is speaking to the soldier in French now. I turn to Tito. And Wendy. We are all here. Still in one piece. There is no greater feeling than coming to the edge and knowing this is not the absolute end after all.

But the danger is not yet past.

I wake up from a dreamless sleep and survey my surroundings. A glistening white streams through the window on my right. It is a princely morning in Kinshasa, the morning after mutinied soldiers ransacked our home and almost killed us.

"They've taken everything," Tito is telling me.

We go through the bullet riddled corridor, watching our steps as we try to walk past broken glass and toppled ceramic vases. There are droplets of blood on the floor and blood splatter on the wall opposite the entrance to the living room. In the living room, nothing is recognizable anymore. The wall aquarium wasn't broken; it was totally pulled out. Where blue water and playful fish should be, there is a large rectangular hole through which one can see the foyer that goes into the kitchen. Dad's super loud music system is gone. Some of his CDs are on the floor, shattered. Bob Marley's smiling visage and dreadlocks are still recognizable from a tiny disc fragment. There's the 1993 Peter Justesen catalog on the shelf, largely untouched. The TV is still there too, broken on the floor, a few inches from its former resting place. Its electric cord, taut, is still plugged into the wall. The settees are gone. The curtains. Even the water closet toilets. I'm left wondering how they were able to uproot so much in one night. And how they were able to bear these things away.

We have no food, no water, and no clothes. Embassy files, Dad's off-white Peugeot 505 with the musical horn he installed to make us laugh anytime he came home, shoes, clothes, suits, slippers ... all gone. I remember our dogs,

Sasha and Maiden, with a crushing feeling of vertigo: I had not considered them during our ordeal. I wonder if they are anywhere to be found. A man in a red cap comes through the black gate, and my father goes out to meet him, and then comes back after a while to find Mummy. "It's time to go," he says. He is still in his pajamas—the only item he can claim as a property. My mother nods her okay and takes us all into the room to change into some clothes that had escaped the soldiers' gaze.

In a moment, we are out under the foreboding sun, gathered in the compound by our black gate. Mummy, Tito, Wendy, Uncle Bernard, Sumbu, and some men—including the man with the red cap, who is now telling my father that we are lucky, because the French ambassador was killed in his home.

I turn around to look at the house that had held us all this time. The first home we had moved into when, three years ago, back in Nigeria, my father received an official letter from the Ministry of Foreign Affairs, informing him that he had been posted to China. We were excited. China was Bruce Lee and cool martial arts. But our excitement was short-lived because he came back with a new letter: the Ministry has changed its mind and posted him to some country in central Africa I hadn't heard of—Zaire.

Dad is barefoot. Mum has Dunlop slippers on, as do Tito and I. Mum whispers to us that we have to find a way to the embassy, where she promises we will be safe. Our bodies are shifting restlessly. The sky is crackling with the energy of apocalyptic endings. If we weren't in it, what we just experienced the night before could make a great adventure movie. We are scared, but we cannot stay here. Outside the black gates, beyond this poor facsimile of a barrier, on the streets littered with corpses, thick columns of black smoke and yelling, are men with guns who would take our lives given the chance. How do we make our way through the lot? What lies beyond this fence?

A path breathes open, snaking into the congress of bowing tall grass. We are quiet, the whole world is quiet. It is just the sound of our labored breathing and, sometimes, the sound of my father's Yoruba and my mother's Yoruba. After what feels like hours, we come to a clearing and scattered homes in small shacks. A flimsy plank of wood has been laid across a gutter for easy passage. Dad helps Mummy walk across, and then he guides me halfway, but I lose my balance as I step off the plank, falling to the ground and scratching my right foot on a stone. I can see the white of my flesh under my black skin, peeled back like a potato under a knife. My dad rubs his hand in my hair, saying sorry, and urging me to keep moving.

We get to the clearing I recognize. We've made it, we must look quite a sight to some car owners—a few of them stare at us as they drive past. There are many cars on the road, and those brave enough to drive have one foot pressed down hard on the throttle. Down the road, across a few sidewalks, there's an avenue of trees, the white-tiled, green-roofed building sits in wait, seemingly undisturbed by the commotion of the last hours. A buff security man swings the door open upon seeing my father, and we step into the clean premises—out of breath, our feet sore from running. The Nigerian flag flutters in the wind, welcoming us to our new home. For now.

*"Maybe being in exile is part of what it means to come home and being at home is a preparation for exile."*

Justice is awkward. Awk-ward. Not forward. "For-words" speak of gold-plated futures in wait. "Awkwards" take note of something else. A Middle English word for clumsy, backward, or perverse was *awk*. The word itself invokes the idea of things lacking a certain grace about them, being of many minds as opposed to walking resolutely in one direction. In spite of the many negative connotations attached to the idea of being awkward, awkwardness is a profusion of grace, and not the absence of it. When we don't know what to say or what to do or where to go, it is often because many paths are open to us, many possibilities are known, and many agencies are making themselves heard. The tip of the tongue is a diving board into finer waters.

This is how things move. *Awkly.*

To make a new world, to move it, to wipe the slate clean, to start again, to retell the stories of the injustices and exclusions and untimely death and soiled seas—what a heady and ravishing proposal!

The awkward thus softly beckons us into a playground so animate and dense with cross-cutting trajectories and unbelievably intricate activity that drawing a straight line from here to there is impossible.

We never begin at the beginning. We always begin at the place already massaged by footfalls aplenty, by sighs embedded in loamy layers of earth, nightly negotiations and strange rituals and spilled blood and muffled sounds and startling textures and painful interpellations, and the budding promise of continuity.

*Bayo Akomolafe says his most sacred work is being present for his family. Born in Nigeria then transplanted to Zaire, a country known for cronyism, corruption and ethnic violence, Akomolafe lost both his home and father at an early age. To address his experience of trauma and civil unrest, he became a clinical psychologist and an advocate for peace and social justice. A clinical psychologist, Akomolafe serves as the Executive Director of The Emergence Network, and lectures at Pacifica Graduate Institute. This essay was adapted from* These Wilds Beyond our Fences, *published by North Atlantic Books and reprinted with permission.*

# CHAPTER EIGHT

## The Dance of Exile

### By Biljana Lipič

In *The Great Work of Your Life*, Stephen Cope considers what Jung called the night sea journey as "… the journey into the parts of ourselves that are split off, disavowed, unknown, unwanted, cast out, and exiled to the various subterranean worlds of consciousness … The goal of this journey is to reunite us with ourselves. Such a homecoming can be surprisingly painful, even brutal. In order to undertake it, we must first agree to exile nothing."[17]

I come from a country that doesn't exist anymore. When my family and my native Yugoslavia were broken into pieces by a brutal civil war, I was exiled from my soul. This is the story of my healing, and how I learned that home is nowhere and everywhere because we carry it in our wild hearts.

I was born in Sarajevo, a 15th-century town in a valley that long ago was at the bottom of the Pannonian Sea. Built by the Ottoman and the Austro-Hungarian empires, this city has long stood at the crossroads of Eastern and Western culture. A meeting place for Christianity and Islam, it has been a place of cross-fertilization and conflict. The shooting of Archduke Franz Ferdinand here in 1914 set off World War I. During the next war, Yugoslavia was divided by the Nazis, and the army was run by the people—paving the way for a new Socialist state.

In the 1970s, my family lived in a blandly modern neighborhood, in a functional flat with two spacious rooms. But the old town had a different flavor, with beautifully crafted buildings, pedestrian walkways, shops and cafés, churches, and mosques.

Both of my parents had known the trauma of war. A teacher and librarian, my mother also battled cancer and lived in fear of its return. My father, an engineer, was a creative genius who was rarely home. Over time, he turned into an alcoholic. One day he started to build an energy-saving house for us in the countryside—a sustainable dwelling way ahead of its time—but he never finished it.

Despite their difficulties, my parents loved me, and encouraged my creativity. My mother let me paint pictures on the doors of our wardrobes and on our kitchen tiles. When my father was around, he showed me how washing machines, radios, and other appliances worked, then taught me how to develop photographs, in our small, window-less bathroom. Following in his footsteps, I built model houses and studied physics. In school I was at the top of my class, and took part in singing and poetry competitions. But, my most private world–where I existed only for myself—was dance.

As my parents' marriage became a battleground, I took refuge in the fields and forests above Sarajevo, walking among the horses and the grazing sheep, gathering mushrooms and wild strawberries, and watching my grandmother make bread. I dreamed about the Serbian Robin Hood called

Novak, who was said to hide in the distant mountain caves. I had another refuge on the banks of the river Tisza with my Crazy Aunt Mira and her family growing vegetables, tending goats, fishing, and hunting wild game.

In 1992, another war appeared on the horizon. Not wanting to fight, my father went into hiding and my mother went numb with fear. With danger in the air, it was hard for me to concentrate on my architectural studies. Just minutes before the start of a long and bloody conflict, I left my homeland, leaping across the giant mountains that had guarded me in my youth, into the unknown.

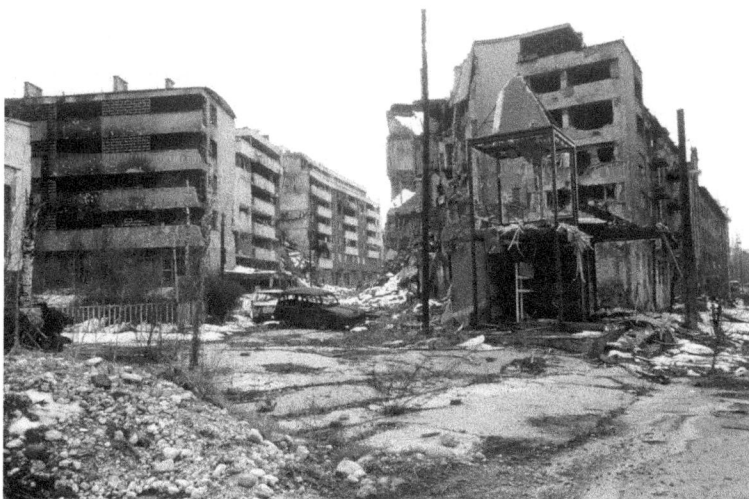

Sarajevo ruins during the Bosnian War.
*By LT. STACEY WYZKOWSKI - www.dodmedia.osd.mil, Public Domain,*
*https://commons.wikimedia.org/w/index.php?curid=1388240*

I landed in London, where I repressed my guilt and shame for leaving those I loved behind, and watched, powerless, as the war destroyed my country and my family.

Yet, my animal instincts pushed me to survive. After finishing my studies, I launched a successful design practice—but I was magnetically pulled back to dance, becoming a pioneer of Argentine tango on this side of the ocean. I opened a club in the dungeons of The Dome in North London, founded an innovative theatre group, and appeared on popular TV programs and in films. In time, I developed an incredibly rich network in the arts and set up dance groups all over the United Kingdom.

From a shy and introverted young girl, I had transformed into a performer on the world stage, known for a visionary way of teaching. Though I was involved in many wonderful creative projects, somewhere along the way, dance had become a drug that allowed me to forget. And, like the girl in *The Red Shoes*, I danced with such abandon that I lost myself.

Juggling many different jobs, traveling the globe with tango as my passport, I had turned my daily life into a marathon. More and more, I felt like a stateless stranger. I was physically and emotionally exhausted, yet the challenges kept building up. After the traumatic death of my parents, I developed an autoimmune disease. Following a couple of unstable relationships, and an early miscarriage, I collapsed.

My healing began as I delved deeper into spiritual disciplines, Jungian psychology, Feldenkreis and other somatic practices. I kept searching until I finally landed in the embrace of shamanism, exploring the sacred bee temples. Eventually, I was called to The Path of Pollen. Buried as part of an ancient ritual, I experienced a symbolic death and rebirth. At one point, I felt that all my body cells were on fire and I became a light inside the great womb of the universe.

With this grounding, I began to face my feelings of isolation, disembodiment, and depersonalization, dropping through layers and layers of loss, war, exile, and intergenerational trauma. In the process, I remembered that I was love and that love was the illuminated darkness, the soul within.

Beyond the need to survive, I was carried by the pure joy of being a part of all that is alive. Here I was more than a dancer—I was the dance itself. From then on, I practiced an actively receptive, sensory, imaginative and erotic way of being—Shamanic tango!—carrying these lessons from the dance floor into every aspect of my life.

In time, I was as fully present, and at home in my body, as I was when I was a child. And when I danced, I noticed the permeable boundary of my own skin, the place where I stop and my partner begins. In this liminal space, I was discovering a unique practice that can take us back to our wild and pristine inner nature. To continue on this path, I left the bustle of the city for the rugged, windswept coast of Cornwall where I set up a new dance studio and began to write about this experience.

Today I live in a houseboat called Floatee on the river Helford, tangoing upon the ocean, moving with the tides, swaying to seasons and the daily shifts in weather. Here I have discovered a simplicity rarely found in the contemporary world. Drawing on all the lessons I learned living in the Sarajevo mountains, I am sparing of resources. I know how to chop wood and make a fire in the stove. I keep a watchful eye on leaks, and air my quarters regularly—the only way to keep clothes free of mold. When the winter cold seeps into my bones, or when storms threaten, I know these challenges are meant to strengthen me, not break me. Over time, nature has become my trusted ally, and Floatee, my sacred twin.

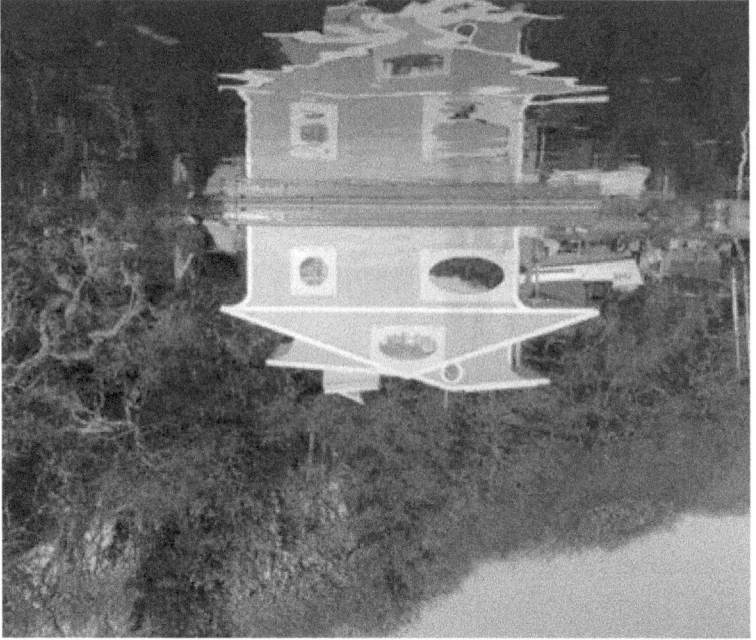

*Floatee, the author's houseboat on the river Helford in Cornwall.*

In our river community, people keep their boats in good repair, clean the plastic from the ocean, and look out for one another. My neighbor, Moni, brings me soup and wildflowers if I am ill. Some nights, I sit by the campfire listening to the soothing voices of the water gypsies, to the musicians and storytellers among us. In the morning, I wake to the sound of the wild children running along the edge of the quay, shouting, "Beeeee, come out to play!" I have become a Crazy Aunt like the one I adored during my childhood summers on the river Tisza.

Floatee is my poetic muse and Cornwall, my healing place. If you come, dear reader, you will gain respect for the deeper, slower rhythms of life. As the tide changes, and Floatee sits on the muddy river floor, you may get in touch with the endless ebb and flow of nature. And by meditating on that which doesn't serve you anymore, you may begin to see yourself as part of the dancing universe. You may even be able to stop time, as you did when you were a child. In the comfort of the silence, you may also begin to see the shape of your own story—and understand its beauty.

As the wonderful John O' Donohue told Krista Tippitt on her PBS Radio program, *On Being,* "Beauty isn't all about just nice loveliness …. Beauty is about more rounded, substantial becoming … (it is) also a kind of homecoming for the enriched memory of our unfolding life."[18]

I remember the town of Sarajevo, the blue mountains of Bosnia, the throbbing city of London, my years of dancing around the globe—and how I landed in the heart of Cornwall. By lovingly giving space to the stories that brought me here, I have slowly freed myself from their grip. Looking with compassion at our lives, we create a sense of sanctuary, then discover layer upon layer of home.

*Biljana Lipič is a Serbian-born multidisciplinary artist, writer and filmmaker, as well as an internationally recognized performer, teacher and choreographer of Argentine tango. She is also the creator of a new, trauma-informed path to embodiment and self-realization.*

..................................................

# Coming Home to the V.A.

## By Andrea Plate

For fifteen years I served as a social worker at the Veterans Administration (V.A.) in Los Angeles counseling soldiers returning from Viet Nam and Iraq—in my care were men and women dealing with multiple addictions, depression, post-traumatic stress disorder, and homelessness. Here I describe the day-to-day problems I encountered at the residential rehab facility known as Domiciliary or the Dom. This is a portrait of a dysfunctional system—one so rule-bound that patients have died in Rehab Facilities, and those seeking help have routinely fallen through the cracks. This raises the disturbing question: How can we expect young people to fight for American values when we fail to provide them with a place of sanctuary when they come home?

In the early years of the Iraq War female veterans slowly trickled in. They, too, were thrust into the general patient pool. Sometimes we had fifty-seven male residents and three females on the same floor. Of course, the women complained that they were "hit on." And they were scared—because their doors had no locks. The open-door policy had been in place for decades, to ensure staff access to all rooms in case of an emergency. Women have served in all of America's wars, but the Veterans Administration did not serve them until the 1980s. Accordingly, when they first arrived at the Dom, we were not prepared. All UAs (urinalysis tests for drugs) for veterans, both male and female, were observed by males on staff. Men observed male patients standing close by, inside the bathroom; they observed female patients from the doorway, facing away, in the direction of the hall.

This practice was not questioned. In fact, once, needing a man on staff to monitor a urinalysis test for a patient who seemed under the influence, the Assistant Chief—Jean, or Ms. Carter, or Sergeant—barked at me: "You can do it yourself! We don't discriminate!" Fortunately, an administrator pulled the tough-talking sergeant aside to explain the ethical and therapeutic ramifications of that:

(1) A female social worker or psychologist cannot watch a man urinate into a cup if she engages him in individual therapy, listens to his deepest confessions, and, as is often the case in individual therapy, becomes the object of his intimate fantasies;

(2) Some of these men have been sexually victimized by women, including their mothers; and

(3) Observations by the opposite sex would open the door to allegations of sexual abuse.

Fortunately, visiting higher-ups issued an immediate ban on the practice of male staffers observing female patients. From then on, only female Domiciliary Assistants (of which there were few) had permission to observe female patients (not too many of those, either, thankfully).

In time, women got their own locks, their own rooms, their own floor at the Domiciliary and their own (female-specific) treatment program. Sexual trauma is a well-known hazard of military service. It had been making news since the Tailhook scandal of 1991, when more than a hundred Navy and Marine officers assaulted or harassed female officers at the Las Vegas Hilton Hotel. Now, with an all-volunteer military, and increasing opportunities for women, staff was directed to trainings on the topic of military sexual trauma, as well as other female-specific treatment needs.

There were a lot of wrongs to be righted, and the V.A. tried to do so all at once, with ferocity. Patient Mary J., for example, came to the program before the implementation of a separate women's track. The vets nicknamed her "Janis Joplin" for her long, straggly blonde hair, ripped jeans and roughhouse ways. One day, she voiced several complaints about "Mr. B."—a thirty-something, African-American veteran who happened to be on my substance abuse treatment team. She said he was "looking at me funny," and she objected to his tone and manner when he said, "You look nice."

This single perceived offense, which Mary mentioned to several on staff, launched a cannonade of phone calls my way: from the women's outpatient clinic at the main hospital; the woman's Domiciliary psychologist; and the Chief of the Dom, who summoned me to her office to ask, "Did you speak to the victim first?"

"No," I explained, defending my decision, "I spoke to my patient (Mr. B), first. He's the one with whom I have a therapeutic rapport. I'm not even sure she was a 'victim.'"

This approach was unacceptable, she said. "Always go to the accuser first!" (Would that apply if the accuser were male?)

From then on I advised my male patients: "Stay away from the women. Don't talk to them. Don't say hi."

One male veteran asked, "When a female smokes a cigarette in the quad, braless, in a sheer blouse, in the freezing cold, am I not supposed to look?" He argued that some of these women, already "messed up" by their military trauma, were actually trolling for sex (then cried foul, maybe to get attention).

Nevertheless, I advised, "Don't look."

It was not an egalitarian culture. It was not a gender-neutral culture. When the laundry machines on the women's hall broke down, female veterans were permitted to use those on the men's floor, anytime, unannounced; but when the second-floor washers on the men's floor broke down, male veterans were denied entry to the women's floor without staff escort. The men complained, so I told the Chief of the Domiciliary. Her answer, "You can tell them that's because of thousands of years of oppression!"

Another example: Women, but not men, were routinely granted weekend passes to go off grounds. When questioned, the Chief said, "They have children!" And men don't?

Now the male veterans' rights were at risk.

Something was wrong; I could sense it, and see it, the moment I returned to work Monday morning when a group of veterans seemed very upset.

"How was your weekend?"

"Lousy!" Something wrong? "You bet!"

Unbeknownst to me, a directive had been issued Friday afternoon that all male veterans were to be "educated" on the topic of sexual harassment. Audrey was assigned to speak to the guys on my floor. She was a "lifer"—the term for those whose only employer was the V.A. She had in fact started there more than twenty years before, in a low-level clerical job. Now she was supervisor of the Dom Assistants. Audrey cut an imposing figure. At 5´11˝, not counting the four-inch stilettoes, the vets described her as "ghetto chic," "hard-ass" or "the African queen." This Monday morning, they vented at what she had "taught" them:

(1) Never look a woman directly in the eyes, because that's intrusive; focus instead on her forehead; and

(2) Never let a woman know you're staring at her from behind. (Audrey told them, "I know when I walk out of this room you're all staring at my ass.")

"What did I think?" the guys asked. "On the contrary," I said, "the eyes are the windows to the soul, so look deeply within." When asked if I, too, felt the heat of their eyes "from behind," I made fun of myself, as I knew they saw me—a skinny uptown girl with a boney butt.

In the early Obama years, the rights of transgender persons to serve in the military wasn't even a hot topic on cable news, or in classrooms and living rooms.

Thus, we were not prepared for Ella Love, a forty-something veteran transitioning from male to female. She was flighty and outwardly girlie, with peroxided hair, a heavily pancaked face and a penchant for floral print, diaphanous dresses. A free spirit, she was prone to cartwheeling down the hall and blowing bubbles during groups on stress management. Anatomically, however, she remained male; her surgery was not yet complete.

Where to house her? First, she was placed on a men's floor, but soon after she complained that the men were "coming onto me." And yet, they couldn't place her on a women's floor. This had been tried a year earlier, with another male-to-female transgender veteran, and resulted in a legal judgment against the V.A. In that case, a female roommate, a survivor of military sexual trauma, claimed she was re-traumatized one night upon awakening to see her transgender roommate in the bathroom, genitalia exposed.

Administrators were so desperate, they considered housing Emily on the "cancer" floor. Emily did not have cancer but the unspoken assumption, or hope, was that these ill veterans wouldn't have the wherewithal to bother her. Then a nurse practitioner strongly objected, "Those cancer patients need peace and quiet, not the belle of the ball!"

Eventually, Emily got a single room. Problem solved.

I didn't know Emily, but I loved Cardi P., also a male-to-female transgender veteran. Her birth name was distinctly masculine—something like Bill Hughes—which was still the name on her patient record. Three times she came to the Domiciliary, tired of homelessness and turning tricks.

The first time she looked predominantly male, dressed in black leather pants, a colorful print bandana and two over-sized silver hoops dangling from her ears. I remember seeing her for the first time, in a heated argument, snarling and stomping away from some macho guys. A short time later, she tested positive for crack and left the Domiciliary program.

I saw her again about a half-year later, waiting to be interviewed for Domiciliary admission. This time she wore a shoulder-length, blonde wig and a baby-blue spaghetti-strap dress, despite the chill of winter. Again, she left the program shortly after coming in.

The third time was the charm—for me, and for Cardi

P. She got her own room on a men's floor. This time, her appearance was far more feminine. She wore dresses every day, wigs in a variety of styles (tousled red tresses; a chic, black bob), and always a velvet ribbon choker, she explained, "to hide my Adam's apple." But her sexual reassignment surgery had been stopped. With an enlarged heart from abusing crack, she was prohibited from further surgeries until she stayed sober, which is what brought her back for treatment.

This girl had moxie. Three mornings a week she strode proudly, if not defiantly, through the sixty men assembled for morning community meetings, always sitting up front. She appreciated not being bothered by the male vets (this time they stayed away, not certain where she stood on the gender spectrum). But at the same time, she was lonely. "I'm the only one of my kind," she once remarked.

Cardi and I built a strong therapeutic tie. She had a history of clashes with staff and was the butt of jokes by those who had previously worked with her. I defended "my girl." I taunted them: "Hey, aren't we supposed to be an empathic therapeutic community?" That stopped them.

To me, this veteran was fun. "I have nothing to wear!" she would say, rolling her eyes in mock exasperation. She gloried in girlish clothes, and they were very flamboyant— one day, a Scottish plaid micro mini from a thrift shop called Out of the Closet; the next, a neon-yellow spandex cat-suit and four-inch strappy stilettos in which she teetered around managing, somehow, not to fall. "Looks like a pineapple!" whispered a woman on staff when she whisked by. Cardi heard that remark. I could tell, by how forcefully she whipped her head away, but at heart she was undeterred.

Cardi was through with suffering. She wanted fun, and she pursued it with a vengeance. She wasn't one to slouch on a bench smoking cigarettes, waiting for the bus with the guys. She was the one beside them, grinding her hips and mouthing the words to a song blasting through headphones. This girl wasn't going to waste a minute!

And she never took herself too seriously. She laughed in fact, telling me about the drug-sniffing German Shepherd that stuck its cold, wet nose up her towel as she stepped out of the shower, still dancing to a Supremes song. It was 7:00 p.m. and the dogs were part of a surprise drug raid underway. Said Cardi, hand clasped over her heart with melodramatic flair, "What a shock!" Then she sang a few bars: "Stop! In the name of love!"

Unlike other vets, she was fearlessly honest, at least with me. She talked about the stepfather who beat her for "acting feminine," and how she had been "born with a flick of the wrist." She explained that in her teens she thought, "I'm just not sexual", and in her twenties "tried" to be heterosexual but "didn't like it." She spoke about the deep personal isolation she felt at having to hide her sexual orientation while in the Service, long before "Don't ask, don't tell."

Despite all this, she was not embittered. Winsome, yes—"I'll never have the jaw… or the hands and feet [of a woman]," she said. Enraged, yes, when decrying the traumas of life as a "trannie" (her term): "It's all about how you look, your face, your body, who looks better than who!" She said it was worse than competition between heterosexual women, "because of all that testosterone and violence." But embittered, no.

Unfortunately, Cardi tested positive for cocaine, as she had twice before, and went AWOL one night. No note, no phone call— typical relapse behavior. I missed her, especially that first day, when I revisited her room, wigs still nailed to the wall, glittery, strappy stilettoes and velvet chokers strewn over the floor.

About a year later, I ran into her at OPCC, the Ocean Park Community Center, a hub of homeless services and temporary housing in Santa Monica, near the beach. She seemed happy, with new therapeutic ties and a sense of acceptance. Heading down the hallway with a laundry basket, she cheerfully greeted residents and staff. But a year after that, she telephoned to ask me about returning to the Dom. "I need help," she said. "I need a connection."

When Cardi came to my office she did not look well. Her hair was matted and tucked beneath a baseball cap. She was hunched inside the folds of an old, faded pea coat. I explained that the Dom had changed, and that all patients now faced a thirty-day restriction to V.A. grounds. She declined, obviously still on crack and unwilling to stop.

I haven't seen Cardi in years. I hope she's alive, but when high-risk patients stop showing up, I always wonder. In recent years, the V.A. has made some advancements in caring for transgender veterans. They not only get their own rooms, but are respected members of the gay—or, to be politically correct, non-normative gender—community. Cardi would have had an easier time.

I am grateful to Cardi for some measure of enlightenment. She showed me, with far more specificity and candor than any academic or clinical course, that gender can often be a state of mind. She had the clothes, the mannerisms, and more *joie de vivre* in being female than many of us who were born that way.

*This chapter was adapted from* Madness: In the Trenches of America's Troubled Department of Veterans Affairs, *published by River Grove books. Andrea Plate was a Senior Social Worker at the West Los Angeles branch of the U.S. Department of Veterans Affairs, within the Veterans Health Administration (VHA), for almost fifteen years. She now teaches "Gender and the Military" at Loyola Marymount University in Los Angeles. As a child actress (Andrea Darvi), she appeared on many television shows during the Golden Era of Television, including* Combat! *and* I Spy.

# CHAPTER TEN

## Pandemic Dreams—Horrors or Healers?

### By Valerie Andrews

In the early days of the 2019 coronavirus pandemic, we lived in constant fear of illness and contagion. It was hard to feel safe in our own beds for our dreams were yet another gloss on the trauma we were experiencing in our daily lives. Sheltering in place, we were in a constant state of "fight or flight." Life under lockdown was a kind of waking dream, calling up our worst anxieties. In the first months of the pandemic, we felt threatened on every level—by other people, by our surroundings, and by nature itself—for this disease had slyly jumped from bats to humans, crossing firm genetic boundaries. To find out how people were coping, I turned to Harvard psychology professor Deirdre Barrett, who collected over 8,000 pandemic dreams and compared them to those after the attack on the World Trade Center on September 11, 2001.

"Back then people dreamed that they were out going about their business then suddenly a plane crashed into the side of a building," Barrett said. "These dreams often incorporated one of the visual elements shown on TV—a plane, a falling building, hijackers with knives. Our pandemic dreams were different because the virus itself was invisible. There was no single dramatic image that everyone was reacting to." In the first stage of the epidemic, people began dreaming about body sensations—having trouble breathing, spiking a fever. Some borrowed dystopian imagery from the endless films they streamed online: "I'm on a street with huge piles of trash, in a scene from *Contagion*."

Insect dreams were common, too. Our fear of being attacked by the virus was represented by angry bees and hornets, a swarm of black flies, a room filled with loathsome bugs. "There were also scenes of worms on the ground and armies of cockroaches," Barrett said. "One woman dreamt about a giant grasshopper with vampire fangs."

The Netflix documentary, *Tiger King,* inspired a dream about the grim realities of unemployment during the pandemic. "A man dreamt he got furloughed and the only job he could find was working for Joe Exotic," Barrett reported. "In the show, employees had to live in hovels and eat food from Walmart's discard bin. The animals and the people weren't treated very well."

Early on, Barrett worried about her students—psychiatric residents working in the hospital emergency room were exposed to the virus on a daily basis. She even dreamed about trying to protect her cat from the virus. As a way of coping, she began making collages like the one below, of a woman carrying a lamb to safety—both of them in gas masks. Working with dream images in a creative way helped her transform that anxiety and begin to cope with her surroundings.

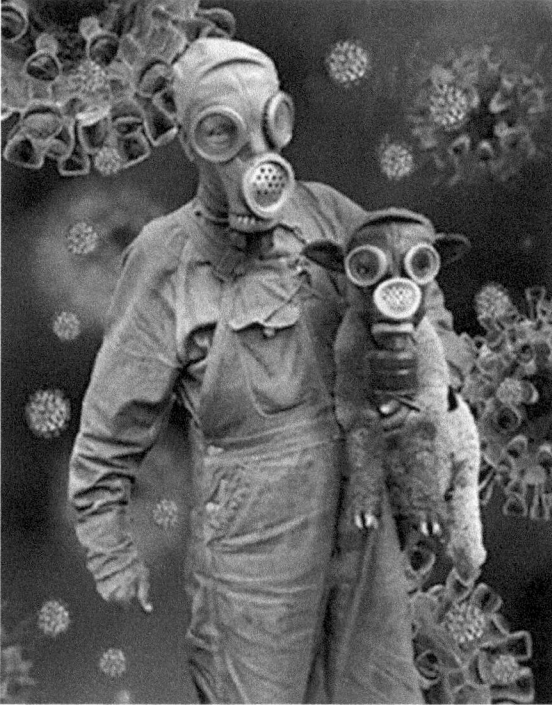

*Art by Deirdre Barrett*

As the months wore on, Barrett continued to focus on dreams during the trials of lockdown. "People sheltering in place alone tended to dream about being imprisoned," Barrett told me. "Those with families dreamt that a bunch of strangers had moved in. One woman, who was home-schooling her only child, dreamt the whole class showed up on her doorstep." Parenting during "shelter in place" was more demanding than ever and our dreams indicated that.

Later in the pandemic, our dreams took an interesting turn, and began to offer images of hope and reconciliation. "Mad Maxx post-apocalyptic dreams were followed by an idyllic scene where people lived together in harmony, finding new ways to cooperate," said Barrett. Then came dreams of whales and dolphins. "These creatures started showing up in ponds or swimming pools in the dreamer's backyard," she added, "In one dream, the whales have learned to fly."

A wholesale clearing of the earth emerged as a major theme, and Barrett cited dreams like this one as evidence: "The dreamer walks into her backyard and sees tall mountains in the distance. She calls her mother and asks how this is possible. Her mother says they have been there all along. 'You just couldn't see them because of the pollution.'"

"In many dreams, the rivers that run through major cities are filled with tropical blue water," Barrett found. "Magical things are happening. The air and water are cleaner. In short, we're getting a glimpse of a better world."

How do we explain these images of regeneration?

"The dreaming mind is older than the waking mind and has a broader bandwidth. It simply knows more," said psychologist Meredith Sabini, founder of the Dream Institute of Northern California in Berkeley. "It has access to survival strategies—ones that have evolved for over two million years."

When I asked about these dreams of planetary renewal, Sabini referred to the principles of evolutionary psychology. "We're longing for a way of life we used to have, in small clans, as hunter-gatherers," she said. "This is how we managed for 99 percent of our history as a species—by living close to the earth. I think our dreams are trying to bring us back to that baseline, to reconnect us to nature and to our original sense of home."

As the coronavirus unfolded, Sabini held a series of online dream workshops. One woman shared this dream:

I'm talking to people about the painstaking and careful work scientists do to learn more about the world. Then a trickster interrupts us, and says, 'Yes, but what about the accidents, and the unexpected, and all the messing up?' I'm then in my old classroom, a naturalist's lab. I have set up a bug terrarium but there's a plant growing in it, with a few small buds. It's comfrey. The trickster knocks the buds off. I decide to save them. They might even be a cure for covid.

"We talked about the word comfrey and this woman's need for comfort," Sabini said. "But there was a bigger message here as well. This dream is about two possible approaches to the pandemic. One involves collecting scientific data and the other, making room for the mysterious and inexplicable forces at work. We need to be open to other ways of looking at the world because the unexpected does happen and could lead to innovation and new forms of creativity."

My own dreams followed a similar trajectory. In March 2020, I was working on a new issue of *Reinventing Home,* a magazine that explores our need for sanctuary, when I came down with all the classic covid symptoms—high fever, fierce headache, dry cough and delirium. For two weeks, I could barely drag myself out of bed. Though fatigued and out of breath, I kept pushing myself to meet an impossible deadline. At this point, I had the following dream: I'm trying to get to an important meeting, but the subway station is closed. It's an arduous walk, and when I arrive, the office is in chaos. Armed men are taking all of my workers into custody. There's a shoot-out and our lives are in danger.

The message was clear: I had reacted to the pandemic with a knee-jerk response, "If I just work harder, everything will be all right." Yet, things weren't going back to normal, and my constant pushing only made me more susceptible to infection. "Deadlines" also proved an impediment to a full recovery. I continued to push until I collapsed.

A second dream, however, provided a strong antidote: A Bengal tiger is walking down the middle of main street. This magnificent animal roams freely through the town—its fur gleaming, its muscles rippling. The creature is one-in-itself. It has no agenda but to simply be.

When I shared these two dreams, Sabini said, "Your fear of being stopped in your tracks came up in the first dream. At that point, you were taken down by the virus. Then, in the tiger dream, your psyche gave you what shamans refer to as a power animal—a guide to your healing process. How do you plan to draw on it?"

"This animal is wild," I responded. "It hasn't been trained to jump through hoops or perform in a circus. There's no way to hold this tiger! Its energy is immense. It has the reservoir of strength I need in order to regain my health."

"Since the virus struck, we've all been holding our breath, waiting to see what will happen next," Sabini added. "The tiger dream is telling you to focus not on deadlines but on maintaining your own life."

After this enlightening conversation, I began to think about the biological purpose of dreaming and why our pandemic dreams seemed to come in pairs. First, a terror dream that alerted us to the physical danger. Then, a second dream that showed us how to cope. But how, exactly, do body and the mind begin to work together? And is there some way we can facilitate this process?

To explore the energetic content of pandemic dreams, I turned to Robert Bosnak, a Jungian analyst who created a technique called Embodied Imagination®. This involves "running an image through the body" to see what physical changes it produces. Bosnak's method has been used by the Royal Shakespeare Company, applied to medical research, and used in psychotherapy practices around the world. The premise: If we work with an image physically, we amplify its power—then it has the capacity to alter our whole organism.

During the pandemic, Bosnak hosted an online group called The Spooky Dreams Café. Here, people learned to create "a personal remedy for living in the pandemic age." The week I joined the group, I heard some fascinating dreams—one about encountering a lion in a swimming pool, another about losing a grandmother's house, and a third about facing the end of the world. Yet, in each case, the dream scenario shifted, leading to an unexpected transformation. The lion turned out to be a reassuring presence. The grandmother's backyard was now a shelter for a strong and stalwart rhinoceros. And as the world was about to end, the dreamer and her family were saved by a giant bird.

Bosnak then asked these participants to channel their dream images through their bodies—to experience the tension at the start of the dream, noting how they felt as their "helper" animals appeared. The change in their comfort level was dramatic. When I focused on the imagery in my own pandemic dreams, I was astonished by the physical transformation they produced. As I recalled the scene of the armed men in my office, my body went rigid, and my heart rate skyrocketed. When I focused on the tiger in my second dream, the muscles in my neck and back relaxed, my heart rate slowed, and I felt thoroughly at ease. I had experienced what the poet Wendell Berry called "the peace of wild things," and wondered: Could our dreams be telling us how to counteract our fears and reach a place of calm and safety?

Bosnak believes somatic dreamwork changes the immune system, and he draws on the emerging science of psychoneuroimmunology to explain how this works. "We believe that the further we move away from habitual consciousness, the closer we come to the autonomic nervous system, our basic Operating System. In computers the OS interacts directly with the motherboard. In humans, this is the place where the image and physical body interact."

My dream with the threatening men hijacking my office triggered a "fight or flight" response. But in the months to come, I would counteract that body terror by drawing on the contained energy of the tiger. Often that meant getting up from my desk and walking languidly through our deserted town, feeling the ripple of the muscles in my back and noting the soft, slow rhythm of my breath. The cure for "my covid complex" was embodying this dream animal and returning to a state of nature. In essence, I was given a prescription that released me from my pre-covid workaholic state. It is a directive I am following to this day.

Our worry about the virus—and about the general uncertainties of daily life—clearly placed the immune system on red alert As we learn to pay attention to our dreams, we can begin reverse that "fight or flight" response.

Somatic dreamwork is a valuable tool that can help us take responsibility for our wellbeing—and begin feel at home within the body of the world.

*Valerie Andrews is the editor of this anthology and the founder of the digital magazine,* Reinventing Home: Culture, Creativity and Character. *She has kept a dream journal for over 50 years.*

PART III

# A NEW STORY
# OF HOME

..................................................

# CHAPTER ELEVEN

# At Home in America—What Myth Now?

## By Thomas Singer

In the past few years, we have been through a pandemic, economic collapse, ever-deepening division, racial violence, floods, and wildfires that have felt apocalyptic. Americans of all stripes have been in a state of great distress, wondering what the future will hold—yearning for a vision, new or old, that will help resolve what I term "cultural complexes" that divide us on issues of immigration, race, gender, abortion, health care, the relationship between rural and urban populations, between the individual and the broader community, and our views on the role of government today.

The profound fault lines that have been growing in our country for several years inspired my book, *Cultural Complexes and the Soul of America*, exploring the many narrative threads that have contributed to the fragmentation of our old mythologies. As a Jungian psychoanalyst, I have a deep interest in the underlying stories of our culture—and the many movements from feminism to gay rights to civil rights to economic and healthcare reform that have surfaced in our new national narrative. We anxiously hope for the emergence of a new guiding vision of who we are and who we want to be as a people going forward.

Anselm Kiefer's sculpture, *The Breaking of the Vessels,* wrestles with the awful intersection of myth and politics in the Nazi era, placing it in the context of the Jewish creation myth of the Kabbalah, in which the oneness of the creation is shattered into many pieces. Kiefer references Kristallnacht, the infamous night in November 1938, when the Nazis smashed the windows of Jewish owned stores. Shards of glass spill onto the gallery floor in Kiefer's sculpture. In recent times, many have felt as though the "oneness" of the United States' democracy and constitution was threatened. As in Kiefer's sculpture, critics have been calling for *tikkun*, a healing of the shattered fragments.

In our search for a unifying mythology, it is not just a matter of a campaign slogan such as Donald Trump's "Make America Great Again" or Bill Clinton's "Bridge to the 21st Century." Unlike creating a brand, an authentic unifying myth can take centuries to develop as it wells up from the psyche of many individuals over generations. Who is to say whether such a new or renewed myth for America, or the rest of the planet, will develop any time soon—or whether several competing myths will vie with one another for dominance?

If we are serious about engaging the deeper meanings of our individual and collective lives, it is often best to begin at home by asking probing questions. Who am I as a person? Who are we as a people? Where is our country headed? How do we heal our fractured national spirit and mend the larger rifts between our parties and our citizens? How can we embrace the profound changes in our political, economic, geographic, and even cosmological reality as we awaken to the fact that we are living on a small, vulnerable planet in a vast universe? I have been contemplating these issues ever since Senator Bill Bradley asked me in 1989, "What myth now?"

At that time, I turned to my dream life with that question, and I got the following response: *I am talking to an ancient sage about the meaning of the rapid changes taking place in the world as the millennium approaches. He has his hands on the skull of a black monastic nun from the early Christian era.*

I have been walking around that dream ever since and, in many ways, it is as opaque and compelling to me now as it was thirty-five years ago. Major upheavals marked the early Christian era. Rome was the center of a vast empire that was beginning to crack both at the periphery and at the center. Early Christianity was competing with Mithraism for the allegiance of Middle Eastern conscripts in the Roman army. In Mithraism, a bull, representing strength and fertility, was the focus of elaborate initiation rites.

At critical junctures in human history, when empires are threatened, different mythologies compete until one emerges as dominant—Mithraism vs. Christianity 2000 years ago, Communism vs. Democracy in the 20th century, or the Economic model vs. Ecological model in the 21st century.

In our new millennium, many have already prophesied what is in store for our civilization and planet. They shout at us with enormous conviction, filling our heads with Utopian promises of extended life and leisure, thanks to science and technology, or with predictions of imminent catastrophe due to famine, war, or ecological disaster. As we grapple with the awesomeness of a truly unknown and unenvisioned future, one Jungian analyst's dream and meditation on the skull of a black nun from the early Christian era does not provide any better crystal ball.

But the dream seems to underline the turmoil of a world in rapid transition; and behind it lies a religious mystery in the form of a long dead, black spiritual woman. Why black and feminine? Is this an image of the introverted soulfulness that we so desperately lack in our contemporary culture and politics? Like a monk contemplating a skull in daily religious practice, my "sage" seems to look upon the skull as a reminder that death is always our companion whether we are staring at the death of civilizations or of individuals.

I like to think that whatever new myth or myths emerge, they will be in the category of "recombinant visionary myth." I like the word recombinant because it likens the formation of a living mythology to the biological process by which genes rearrange themselves to create new life forms.

It further suggests that the building of mythology is an evolutionary process whereby bits and pieces of a myth are rearranged to suit changing needs. The Christian story with its claim of a reborn man/God incorporated messianic yearnings and beliefs that had circulated widely in the Jewish faith as well as in pagan religions that celebrated a literal "eating" of the God.

I add the word "visionary" to this process of myth-building to incorporate our emerging view of the cosmos and the relationship between the human, nature, and spirit.

And I also imagine that there will be competing myths vying for our attention for some time to come.

In his essay on *The Cultural Complex and Addiction to Dominion*, Jerome Bernstein zeroes in on our centuries-old belief that human beings have dominion over all creation on earth. He then goes on to describe the emerging paradigm of reciprocity—another recycled view. The primary characteristic of reciprocity as a psychic force, he says, "is a deep spiritual knowing that all life is sacred and, given that tenet, that a healthy life force requires respect for all species and living in balance with all its forms."

He is not speaking about an external belief system but of "a knowing from within the self and between humans and non-human life forms."

In a parallel but different articulation, Betty Sue Flowers frames the Economic Myth as being challenged by the Ecological Myth. She does not dismiss the positive value of the drive for growth and profit. The Economic Myth, she says, fuels globalization which is "necessary in order to solve the most pressing problems of the future, which are global in nature, including climate change, inequality, and rules for the governance of artificial intelligence and biotechnology." But she posits the emergence of the new Ecological Myth as a counterbalance:

> In the Ecological Myth, the supreme value is ... health, or well-being. Health, which comes from a root meaning wholeness ... Here the health of societies and of the planet is not sacrificed for economic growth. We are struggling together as a human species to move into that new myth because it requires an unprecedented level of imagination, cooperation, and transformation.[19]

For some time, I have embraced the emerging scientific myth that climate change has led us to the brink of the abyss in terms of life on the planet. Almost every scientist in the world who studies this phenomenon has come to the same conclusion. But, recently I have returned to the dream of the sage and the black monastic nun of the early Christian era and found my way to this larger ecological story.

When one discovers the myth on an inner level, it leads to a different kind of knowing, less honored perhaps than the "objective" scientific truth. But such an inner experience often has far more impact than a commonly accepted narrative. Although I have embraced the growing reality of climate change and have on occasion experienced the sacredness of the earth, only recently have I felt a deeper awareness of what is happening to the planet. I know that many have come to the inner awareness of the ecological myth long before I have, but for us to take action on a collective level, more of us need to have such a personal revelation.

Our new mythology will emerge, not from political spin doctors, but from the depth of the unconscious. And it is our task to begin listening on that level. That means tuning in to our dreams and looking for the "big ones" that speak to our relation to the culture, and to the value of life itself.

My understanding of my own deep dream has been aided enormously by Jules Cashford, our era's foremost scholar of lunar and Gaia mythology. Indeed, Jules has become the real-life equivalent of the sage who knows something about civilizations in transition and meditates on things that endure the passage of time. I know that the skull of the black, monastic nun of the early Christian era suggests something dark, inner, spiritual, and feminine. I know that

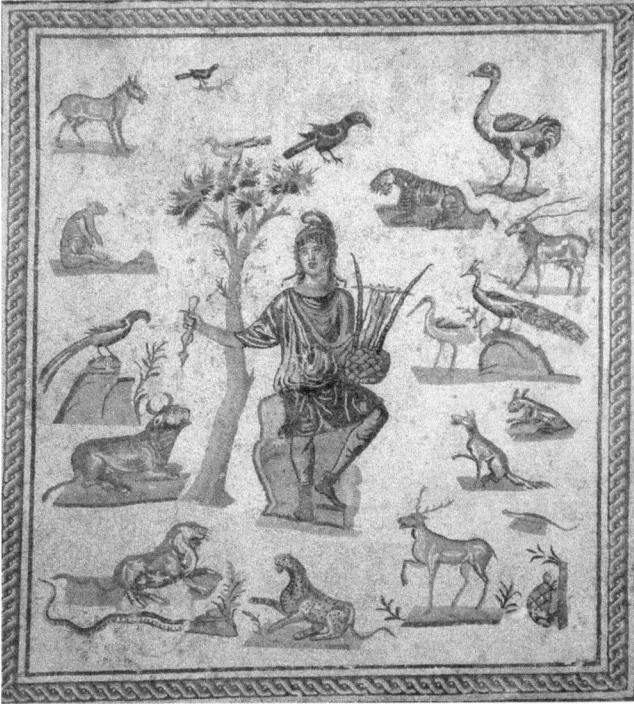

*Mosaic: Orpheus serenading the animals.*
*Foto di Giovanni Dall'Orto - Own work, Attribution,*
*https://commons.wikimedia.org/w/index.php?curid=1303452*

the sage with his hand on her skull suggests that this knowing is "hands-on" and that whatever the skull symbolizes seems to be as true for our era as for the early Christian era. But Jules took an intuitive leap, suggesting that the dark spiritual feminine energy in my dream is lunar. Lunar knowing begins with gazing at the phases of the moon and literally learning to reflect on things in a different light. It focuses on recurring changes—the movement of natural, living processes, of becoming and disappearing, of being born, growing, dying and being born again. And thus it reveals the sacredness of Mother Earth, of Gaia.

Jules then sent me a rare, esoteric image of Jesus from the earliest Christian era. He is on the cross, beneath a crescent moon (indicating rebirth), and the seven stars of the Pleiades. The inclusion of the words "Orfeos Bakkikos" generously embraces other people's gods, in particular honoring the Orphic tradition that celebrated the story of Demeter and Persephone, and the creation of the seasons—the way the year itself progresses from the darkness to the light.

The Jesus of the apocryphal Gospel of Thomas (150 AD) embodied a different kind of wisdom than that which

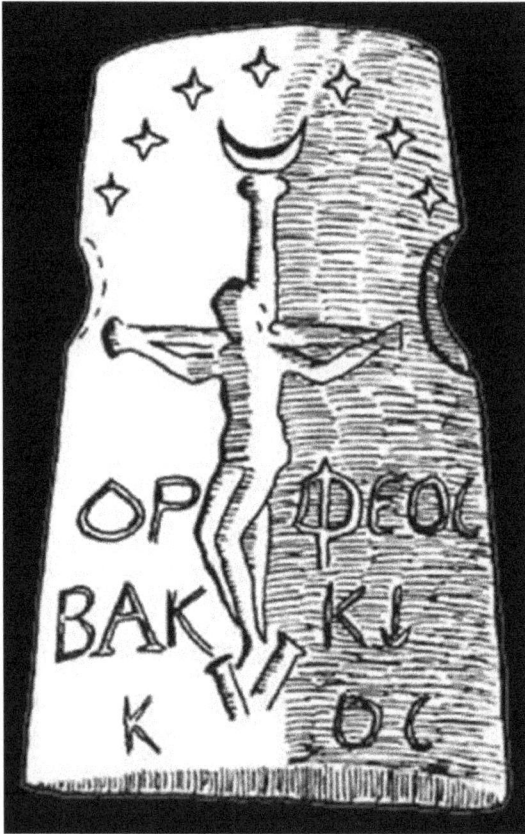

*Image courtesy of Jules Cashford*

was codified in Christianity centuries later. Cashford writes: "The early Christians saw their own Christ in the mythic lunar tradition of the dying and resurrected god of a unified world—in the tradition of Dionysos and Orpheus and the crescent of the Pleiades above, the oldest of whom is Maia the mother of Hermes."[20]

In the beginning, myths are open-handed, generous, and draw unabashedly on other traditions.

In the dream, the sage calls on me to reclaim this early mode of understanding where the Earth is not experienced as "dead" but as living and sacred as is everything else.

What might the skull of the black nun be bringing back to life? As we begin to open to a new myth, it reminds me of a time long ago when another new vision came into the world, of loving one another, and of loving the whole universe as oneself. In the Gospel of St. Thomas, "Jesus said: I am the All. Cleave a piece of wood and I am there. Lift up the stone and you will find me there."

I envision spending the rest of my days meditating on this strange, compelling dream. Jules says there is plenty of good guidance here: "If we take this kind of knowing back far enough, the lunar way of thinking includes darkness and does not oppose it, even finds in the darkness a place of rebirth. The dream sage might be pointing to a new vision of the whole which, looking upon the Earth from beyond the Earth, might have already begun, Earth becoming a 'person'—animate— who deserves a name not just as the ground we tread upon, and put pesticides in. It seems to me that the term *Gaia*, the last time Earth was held to be sacred, is already there."

*Thomas Singer, MD, is a psychiatrist and Jungian psychoanalyst, practicing in San Francisco. He is the editor of a series of books exploring cultural complexes in Latin America, Europe, Asia, Australia, and North America.*

# CHAPTER TWELVE

......................................................

## From Active Imagination to Wildlife Preservation

### By Andrea Wells

In *Inter Views* with Laura Pozzo, James Hillman cautions us not to turn dream animals into symbols of what's going on inside the psyche but to respect them in their own right.[21] This is the story of how I moved from engaging animals in my dreams to helping endangered animals survive by protecting their natural habit.

My fondness for turtles began early in life. I grew up on 20 acres in the Minnesota countryside, in a classic farmhouse that was once a parsonage with an old red barn. The creek in our back pasture had turtles along with frogs, crayfish, and a few catfish. Family vacations to Minnesota's 10,000 lakes offered encounters with snapping turtles, musk turtles and painted turtles all with personalities of their own. I even had a pet turtle, Sam.

At eighteen, I left home and came to the California coast where I began to dream of his distant cousins—deep sea creatures that can live for up to a hundred years: I am holding a baby sea turtle in my hand. I promise to protect it and take it to freedom. As Delmore Schwartz once wrote:

"In dreams begin responsibilities." In a series of dreams, over many years, I discovered my calling to protect these creatures, and to explore the human-animal bond.

Why did these hard-backed reptiles have such a strong appeal? I was a shy young girl in love with nature and spent my time riding horses and exploring the mysteries of the creek, always more at home with animals than people. In social situations, it felt safer not to stick my neck out. I had a natural affinity with the turtle with its retractable head and hidden self. As a child, I'd only known the backyard kind and those who swam in the bathtub of a Midwestern lake, but when I moved to the West Coast I encountered a creature that could grow to be up to 700 pounds, measured 7 meters long, and spent a hundred years beneath the sea.

As I began to think of all the turtles I had known, I had an unusual dream: The turtles are coming up from the depths of my body and trying to get out of my mouth. I know that I must relax my throat and let these turtles out.

This is how turtles became my totem animal. In this initiation, I associated them with the process of finding my own voice—and becoming a passionate advocate for wildlife.

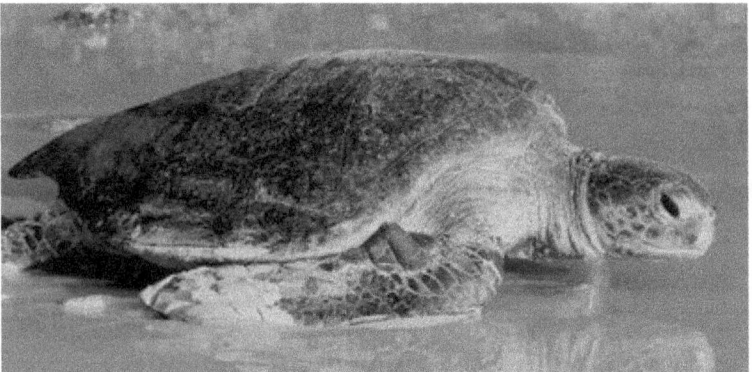

*Sea turtle in the Galapagos, photo by Andrea Wells*

Whale dreams were another story—they were an introduction to awe and wonder. A few years later, when I was studying psychology in Los Angeles, I signed up for a whale watching trip sponsored by Greenpeace. That day, we discovered a dead young whale with fishing line wrapped around its body. This was a sad and shocking experience. Our guides hauled it in for an autopsy so they could make a case against the use of certain fishing nets, and I began to understand that these amazing creatures are in need of our protection. On that same day, gray whales and humpbacks sidled up to the boat, eagerly showing off for us.

When I stepped off the boat, my whole body was quivering, and not long afterward one of these creatures came to me in a dream:

> My room is full of water, and a whale is swimming around in it. She likes it when I scoop up some water with my hands and pour it into her mouth. She has to go to back to the sea, and I worry that, in the transport, she'll be rolled up in a net and treated roughly. Somehow, we get her to the beach and she begins to swim away. I ask how I will recognize her when she comes back again. We both decide we would simply "know" each other.

Over the years, I learned how to dialogue with these dream animals—to actually sit and listen to what they had to say to me—using a Jungian technique called Active Imagination. I tried not to project my own feelings and emotions onto these extraordinary creatures, but to recognize the instincts and affinities we have in common. Animals and people have the same evolutionary history. If we take the time to understand the qualities we share, we become richer, fuller human beings.

Through Active Imagination, I came to know the turtle part of me as a quiet, deep, wisdom, but my dialogue with the whales took more time to come into focus. Whales are the largest animals on the planet and the first world travelers. A gray whale can cover a jaw-dropping 13,988 miles—halfway around the world from Russia to Mexico and back in 172 days. And the blue whale that looks like a steamship in the water, is one of the biggest explorers—logging 16,000 miles in a single migration. They seemed to be calling me to move beyond my comfort zone, to leave the confines of the dreamworld and pursue these relationships into daily life.

In Monterey Bay, California and in the Hawaiian islands, I watched groups of whales, jumping, breaching, and tail flapping, as they gathered for a family reunion. The more I learned about the challenges to their habitat—from fishing boats and shipping lines, from noise and water pollution, the more I wanted to help them flourish. I began supporting the Sea Shepherd organization run by Paul Watson, the former head of Greenpeace. Watson was action oriented. He was given an old rundown boat and started interfering with Japanese whaling ships that claimed to be doing research but were illegally killing whales. Watson was fearless—he got his boat between the whales and the Japanese ships and completely shut them down.

Next, I joined a local rescue team that frees whales that get caught in ropes and nets off the California coast.

Other animals were calling to me, as well. On a research site on the Caribbean coast of Costa Rica, I sat with leatherback turtles that were laying eggs to protect them from nearby poachers. This kind of boots-on-the-ground activism made me feel more alive than ever. I wanted to do more, so each summer I volunteered to work with a wildlife conservation team in South Africa. One of my first projects was de-horning 90 rhinos on the reserve—a drastic but necessary measure to deter poaching and slow the rate of this animal's extinction. Rhinoceros horn is in high demand in Asian countries as medicine and in some, it is a symbol of wealth and power. Poachers hack away at the horn with machetes, crippling the animals, and leaving them to die in agony. It was more "humane" to remove this part of their anatomy and ensure that these endangered creatures would be left alone. Before we began the procedure, I'd place my hand on a sensitive spot behind the rhino's ear and whisper, "I'm sorry this is so distressing. We love you, and we are doing this to help you." Dehorning has lowered poaching rates by 99 percent.

Over the years, this team has freed hyenas and elephants from snares and "translocated" lions, cheetahs, and rhinos—moving the males to new preserves to promote a healthy diversification of blood lines. I think of this hard but rewarding work as the housekeeping we need to do to save the planet and preserve its richness and diversity.

It all comes down to home. The number one threat to wildlife is their loss of home or habitat. While we can help endangered species to survive, there must be enough land to support them. The conservation of wild animals in closed reserves is a complex science. Lion prides must have enough territory to roam, or they will kill each other. Cheetahs need enough area to steer clear of lions. They key is giving each animal the space it needs.

If we encounter certain elephants on a bush road, we put the Jeep in reverse and back up hastily. Sometimes we'll turn around and drive 40 minutes out of our way to accommodate an aggressive bull. The elephant gets the right of way, and that's all there is to it.

We humans are so cut off from our surroundings that we tend to limit our territory to the outline of bodies. Early hunter-gatherers had a much larger sense of their own personal space. They migrated thousands of miles when food sources were low, and, on a daily basis, ran long distances to secure their prey.

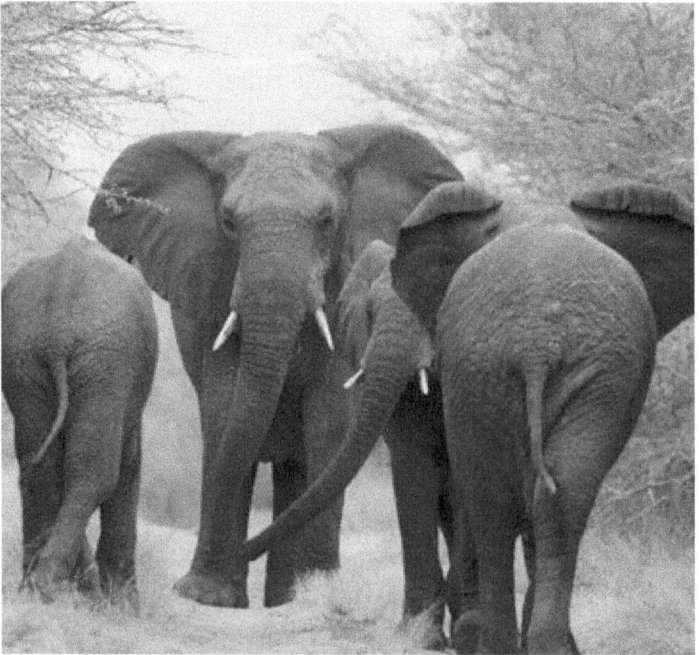

*Photo courtesy of Andrea Wells*

Elephants are constantly on the move and roam even further than we thought. In one reserve, 75,000 acres support 110 of these majestic creatures.

The first thing you learn in the bush is to respect an animal's migration route, water route, mating route. If you start to encroach, believe me—they'll know. It's impossible, for example, to sneak up on an elephant. Their feet have something similar to a whale's sonar that alerts them to invaders. From vibrations in the ground, they can detect the motor of an approaching Jeep or tell what's happening to a herd that's miles away.

In Africa, you begin to rethink your definition of home. Elephants may walk all day long, covering the whole reserve. To find water and food, they can log at least 50 miles a day. Home, for them, is always on the move. That's why they pace back and forth so poignantly when they're locked up in a zoo.

We humans place so much value on putting down roots. For us, owning a home signifies that we have earned our place in the world. It's a rite of passage that indicates we've reached a certain level of professional success. But like the elephants, my home is on the road. Over the years, I've found my place alongside the animals. They've become "my people" and their habitat, my *terra firma*.

There's a deep connection between humans and wildlife—if you spend time in the bush, you will feel it in your soul. Over the centuries, we've poached endangered species, invaded habitats, and destroyed the wilderness. As a consequence, we're disconnected from our own wild nature. When we are disconnected from our own instincts, we suffer emotionally, and spiritually. But there is some serious physical fallout, too.

Zoonotic diseases (illnesses passed from animals to humans) are on the rise because we're invading animal territories. Lyme disease is now attributed to our encroachment on the forest habitat. The coronavirus appears to have come from wildlife poaching—a pangolin stolen from its home in Africa then sold in a Chinese wet market. Tourism in remote areas has brought us into contact with infection-carrying bats.

The question is, how much space will we take over, disturbing natural habitats with our drilling, shipping, trading, building, dumping, and endless power lines? When will we realize that Thoreau was right? "In wildness is the preservation of the world."

Maybe we can take a clue from whales, the first global citizens. In the movie, *Star Trek: The Voyage Home,* whales are the centerpiece of civilization—the whole planet depends on the safety of these beings. In their travels, they weave an invisible shield around the planet. Their idea of home is a cosmic tapestry, an endless skein of thread that transcends countries and corporate identities. If we spend time with these gentle giants, they will help us craft a new cosmology, one in which all life forms are deeply entwined and interrelated.

We need to listen to the animals, get to know them intimately once again. That's why I urge people to get involved in conservation—to donate to their favorite wildlife organizations or volunteer in their local communities. When you are hands-on with animals, you realize that by serving them you're healing something deep within yourself.

These are hard times, and it's easy to feel daunted—to give up hope that we can save the animals and save a portion of this Earth. When I need a jolt of encouragement I think back on my conversation with a whale. "Take more risks!" she said. "Quit beaching yourself! Come out of your comfort zone and dare to do some big things in the world."

*Andrea Wells is passionate about wildlife conservation, wildlife photography, and tulips. She spends two months each year working alongside a wildlife conservation team in South Africa. She has a master's degree in clinical psychology and is a licensed MFT in private practice in Santa Cruz, California specializing in Jungian dreamwork, grief work and discovering the wild soul within.*

# CHAPTER THIRTEEN

...................................................

# Grassland Woman—Understanding Nature's Archetypes

## By Mary Reynolds Thompson

A friend and eco-feminist once told me that she believed American women did not feel they belonged to the land because they were relative newcomers and just coming to terms with their own history. In truth, many of us in the West are waking up to the wounds of colonialism and the horrors of genocide and slavery. Confronted with our brutal past, we can struggle to feel part of the land's in-dwelling spirit. And yet, we must find our way back.

When a culture is disconnected from the land, we grow up with the wrong stories. Author and animist Sophie Strand writes, "I am much more interested in ensoilment than ensoulment. I want to have actual roots."

Nationalism, so-called "love of country," is mostly devoid of care and concern for the land and for the larger Earth community. We swear allegiance to an abstraction while dismissing the values of those who for millennia lived in intimate and reciprocal kinship with the land. Nationalism pumps us up so that we feel ascendant, all-powerful. It forgets that belonging is rooted in humility, from the word humus, meaning "earth." As someone whose lineage includes Irish, English, Scottish, and Romany, and with ancestors who crossed the Atlantic east to west and back again several times, I find it hard to say where I am from.

Like many transplanted people, I feel a sense of bifurcation, of having roots in more than one country. I identify with my birthplace in England but also with my chosen home in California. But does this necessarily stop me from belonging? The world, after all, is made of nomads as well as nesters. We aren't all able to remain in one place. Today, with millions forced by war, famine, and climate disruption to seek refuge in foreign lands, many of us are literally out at sea, in search of a home.

The quest for belonging is complicated and, at times, heartbreaking. It haunts us and hits us in our most vulnerable places. But remember, as you complete this journey you have found a home within yourself. You have learned that belonging is about more than finding the perfect place to settle, it is about embracing an authentic ground of being. Further, you cannot belong if you don't make yourself vulnerable and share yourself with others, honestly and fully. Finally, belonging won't fall into your lap. It flourishes through the practice of sharing, reaching out, connecting, relating, and loving one another.

A Grassland Woman knows that without the earth-worm or the prairie dogs, her own ecological niche would not survive. Every patch of ground has its own community. Every patch of ground offers an opportunity for intimacy, every encounter, a chance for belonging. It takes courage to extend yourself and risk being repelled by some and inconvenienced by others' demands on you. True belonging includes putting up at times with people you sometimes wish would find their belonging elsewhere, or a location that doesn't easily nurture you. And yet, each of us has a place within the larger picture.

I live in Pacheco Valle, a boxed canyon bordered by steep forested hills, north of San Francisco, in a condominium I have shared with my husband for over twenty years. Our neighbors mostly keep to themselves, and we rarely get together to walk or share a meal. Yet this is a place of many wonders. To enter the valley, you pass a large meadow that harbors deer and songbirds and a seasonal creek that spills down one side like a communion veil. This land is a haven for hawks, bobcat, coyote, and field mice. In spring, it is briefly covered in popsicle-bright California poppies. It also hosts the oldest midden, or burial site, 3,000 years old, of the Miwok tribe. About ten years ago, we learned that the meadow was to be sold. The land was zoned for light commercial usage, and the thought of the meadow being blighted with anonymous shops and parking lots galvanized the community. But would the owners (the Gannett newspaper company) sell the land to the Pacheco Valle residents? And for what price? And if we could buy it, could we then donate it to Marin Open Space for public use in perpetuity?

The challenges were immense, but we got a proposition on the ballot that would allow residents of Pacheco Valle to tax themselves in order to purchase the land. My husband and I went door-to-door garnering support for this measure. We met scores of neighbors. After many months of work, everyone playing their part, we acquired the land, and held our first-ever community party. We had come together to preserve a meadow and its unique place in the ecosystem and in our hearts. Our political affiliations didn't matter—only the longing to keep this piece of land intact.

Like the hawk and coyote who share a meadow, the strands of our stories run together. Together, we bear responsibility for the places we make our home. But here's the thing: The land is not only shaped by us, it also shapes us in return. If we refuse to come together protect it, then who will we become in the process? What will we lose? How much less resilient will we be? And if we learn to love it and care for it, what then? What can we do together, what can we become together, that sustains and celebrates a circle of belonging that holds us all?

It is not in the lofty but in the lowly that most of life is lived. In *After the Ecstasy the Laundry,* Buddhist practitioner Jack Kornfield notes that life is comprised of both mundane chores and spiritual adventures. Washing travel-soiled laundry may not be as exciting as the trip itself, but it is an element of it. To hang your clean, mended laundry out to dry on a blustery morning can also be part of your rewilding. We know that the patriarchy undervalues what is called "woman's work": caregiving, cleaning, cooking. These chores are never finished. But if we overlook the value of this repetitive "feminine" work, it's not just our dreams that we dismiss—it is the stuff of our daily lives.

One of the most radical steps you can take as a Grassland Woman, therefore, is to celebrate the cyclical, seasonal work of women. Raising children? Wild work. Caring for elders? Wild work. Tending a garden? Wild work. Founding a company? Wild work. Daily life, whatever form it takes, is not incompatible with wildness; rather, wildness enlivens and refreshes us in our everyday existence. And if we try to live without it, we will tire and fade.

As a Grassland Woman, you delight to nourish and care for that which you love, be it family, community, nature, creative pursuits, causes or whatever wild work draws your nurture. This caring comes directly from your internal sense of freedom. It comes from a place of aliveness deep within your soul. In nourishing, tending, ministering, you are honoring your own values rather than doing what is expected of you. Everyone can sense this. This is how you shift the field of consciousness. This is how you create the ground out of which new life can spring.

The strength of Grassland Woman resides in her thick network of deeply planted roots, the deeper the better. As we come to know her, we begin to build our own tapestries of connection. This is what enables us to survive and thrive, not only in times of plenty but in times of drought. Grassland Woman calls us to bloom in the smallest niches, to put down roots and make connections—even in stony ground. The modern world has made loess (wind-blown soil) of us all.

We are, in the truest sense of the word, rootless. We have been ripped from the Earth. Untethered, we feel increasingly anxious and stressed. Today, virtual reality eclipses the wisdom of our senses, while endless miles of pavement and expanding wireless networks cut us off from the Earth's magnetic energy.

But you know better. As a Grassland Woman, you understand that you are made of the same matter as the Earth, born from her breath, her belly, and her bounty. Beneath the loamy soil is the soft dissolve of your ancestors. In your lungs, the breath of forests; in your blood, the salty oceans; in your bones, the residue of stars. You cannot not belong. It is one thing to know this intellectually, however, and another to live it. So how do we re-learn the art of belonging? How do we repair our severed bonds to this beautiful and still fertile world? The root word for religion, *religare*, means "to bind together."

Awakening to the spirit of Grassland Woman, we recall the umbilical cord that connects us to the greater body of Earth and Cosmos. And thus, the original binding spirit and true purpose of religion is restored. Grassland Woman has a different sense of the sacred than the one most of us were raised with. She reminds us that we were never banished from the garden. We were never told not to eat its fruit or to hide our nakedness. In her creation story, woman did not burst forth from the rib of man. She was birthed from the great womb of Earth and Universe. At this stage of your journey, you are not in exile anymore. You are not cast out from the web of creation. You are not a mistake. You are, my sister, my beloved friend, cherished and wanted. Grassland Woman joyfully welcomes home the prodigal daughter, the adored child of the Earth. The snake and the apple tree, the shivering grasses, and the wild blue creeks embrace you as you return to her fold.

If you can grasp this great love, the love that lies at the heart of belonging, then nothing will ever be the same. Old patterns of shame, blame, judging, and comparing lose their potency. You realize that you were never cast out of Eden. That was the wrong story. And it is being righted and rewritten as you are being rewoven into the fabric of the world. Eighty percent of prairie grasses live underground. Everything that makes you brave and rich with life originates there, too, in this fecund space. Begin by rooting in that tangible reality. Wherever you find yourself, your roots run long and deep. You are the beloved child of the Earth and a long evolutionary process that has given birth to you. Let your song be one of belonging.

*Mary Reynolds Thompson, Founder of "Live Your Wild Soul Story," is an award-winning author, facilitator of poetry therapy, and a pioneer in the emerging field of spiritual ecology. She has created a unique program of transformation based on nature's archetypes, taking us on a journey into the depths of our untamed souls. This chapter was adapted from her book,* The Way of the Wild Soul Woman: 5 Earth Archetypes to Unleash Your Full Feminine Power, *published by Findhorn Press.*

# CHAPTER FOURTEEN

..................................................

# Dialogue on the Mall

## By Joseph J. Ellis

Ask a group of realtors to name the most valuable plot of ground in the United States and they will end up arguing about the price per square foot in Manhattan, San Francisco, and Boston.

Ask a group of historians the same question and they end up agreeing, with scarcely a dissenter, on the Mall and Tidal Basin in Washington, D.C. You can't buy space there. All the permanent residents earned their plots for reasons that defy the measures of the marketplace.

The reasons do not defy the shifting winds of politics. The Jefferson Memorial, for example is located on the Tidal Basin in a space previously reserved for Theodore Roosevelt. His cousin, Franklin Roosevelt, effectively stole the space for Jefferson in the 1930s in order to provide the Democratic Party with a canonized saint who offset Abraham Lincoln, already perched on the Mall as the Republican Party's saint.

Soon after the dedication of the Jefferson Memorial in 1943, a dialogue began between Jefferson and Lincoln over the role of slavery and race in American history. Though the conversation between the two icons occurs at a transcendent level beyond the range of human ears, it is discernible by lip-reading the steady parade of tourists at each memorial as they mumble the words on the marble panels surrounding each rotunda. George Washington had chosen to remain silent during this dialogue. There are no words on the Washington Monument save for the graffiti scrawled on the staircase leading to the top by several generations of tourists.

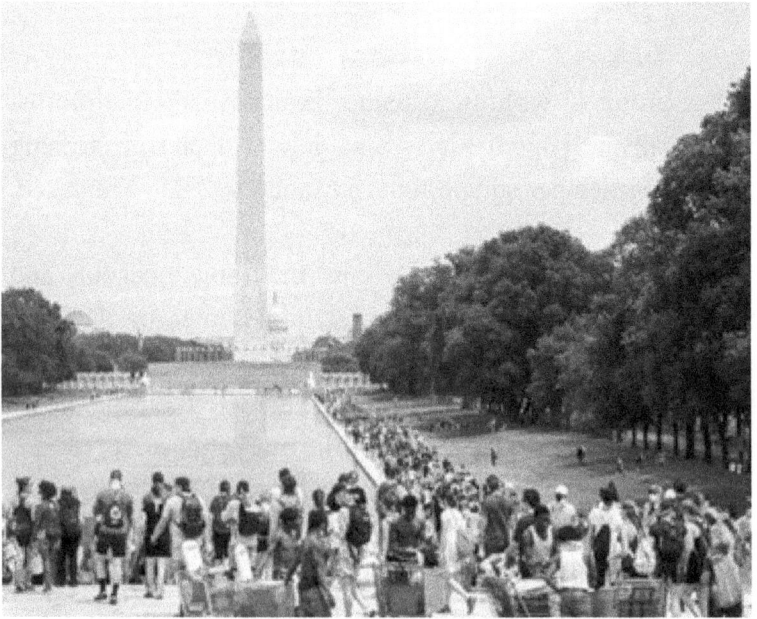

*The National Mall in Washington. Photo by Koshu Kunii on Unsplash*

Here is Lincoln, channeling Jefferson's wisdom in the Gettysburg Address (1863): "Four score and seven years ago our fathers brought forth on this Continent a new Nation, Conceived in Liberty, and dedicated to the proposition that all men are created equal." By speaking those words, Lincoln was declaring that the Civil War was not just about preserving the Union; it was also about ending slavery. He was invoking Jefferson's words in 1776 to keep the promise in 1863 that Jefferson himself had failed to keep during his lifetime as a slave-owning statesman.

But instead of scolding Jefferson for his hypocrisy, Lincoln celebrated him for his visionary view of human equality: "All honor to Jefferson, to the man who had the coolness, forecast, and capacity to introduce into a merely revolutionary document, an abstract truth, and so to embalm it there, that today and in all coming days, it shall be a rebuke and stumbling block to the very harbingers of reappearing tyranny and oppression." One can only imagine Jefferson smiling at the tribute, relishing the irony of "a merely revolutionary document," basking in the glory of crafting the American Creed.

Meanwhile, over on the Tidal Basin, tourists were whispering the words that Lincoln found so inspirational. Here are the magic words of American history: "We hold these truths to be self-evident; that all men are created equal; that they are endowed by their Creator with certain inalienable Rights; that among these are life, liberty, and the pursuit of happiness."

In murmuring the words most tourists resemble members of a congregation in prayer. Jefferson seems to generate an electromagnetic field where "these truths" are articles of faith that all are expected to embrace with unspoken devotion. (If you think about it, that's what being self-evident means.) The Jefferson Memorial serves as a semi-sacred zone where political differences dissolve in deference to transcendent moral principles, a uniquely American version of the Delphic Oracle.

A third voice joined the ongoing dialogue in August of 1963 when Martin Luther King delivered his "I Have a Dream" speech on the steps of the Lincoln Memorial. Though speaking in Lincoln's shadow, King announced that he had "come to collect on a promissory note" written by Jefferson. He was obviously referring to the very words Lincoln had cited to justify the end of slavery, which King now claimed as a mandate to end racial discrimination. This was an expansive version of Jefferson's promise that not even Lincoln had seen fit to propose.

King's voice became a permanent presence on the Mall in August of 2011 with the dedication of the Martin Luther King Memorial. Although King is looking towards Lincoln, his message floats across the Tidal Basin to Jefferson as the primary source for the egalitarian agenda of the Civil Rights Movement.

What the lifelong Virginia slaveholder meant when he wrote the magic words, King argued, was less important than what the words said to us now. The distance that America needed to travel in order to reach the promised land was less important than our collective commitment to racial equality as a goal. Like the arc of the moral universe, the arc of the dialogue on the Mall bent toward justice. The fact that the first Black president in American history was present for the dedication of the King Memorial seemed to indicate that King's dream was coming true.

The exact opposite was occurring. The proliferation of cell phones among the tourists and visitors to the Mall filled the airwaves with voices of disbelief that a man who looked like Barack Obama could possibly be their president. Within the new echo chamber, King's dream was described as a nightmare. White protestors at the King Memorial wearing "Make America Great Again" hats resembled the unique replication of King's head emerging from the mountain as a joke about howling into the wilderness. "Again" for them meant before Barack Obama and before the Civil Rights Movement.

Meanwhile, over on the Tidal Basin, protesters carrying Black Lives Matter signs were calling for the removal of the Jefferson Memorial, describing it as a celebration of both slavery and racism. The panels inside the rotunda, especially the one with the magic words about human equality, were monuments to American hypocrisy by a false prophet.

A panel with the following words from Jefferson's autobiography was, not so mysteriously, missing: "Nothing is more certainly written in the book of fate than that these people are to be free. Nor is it less certain that the two races, equally free, cannot live in the same government." Nature, habit, opinion have drawn indelible lines of distinction between them: For Jefferson, Black inferiority was the most self-evident truth of all. Despite Jefferson's well-earned reputation for duplicity, he was sufficiently candid to play the race card up.

Where does that leave us? Well, the Mall always was, and always will be, a semi-sacred space where Americans come together to meditate, mourn, and remember who we were, and are, as a people and a nation. When the ongoing dialogue confronts the race question; however, the collective consensus breaks down because a sizable minority of white Americans, most of whom would pass a lie detector test proving they are not racists, have never internalized the egalitarian assumptions of the Civil Rights Movement. As a result, the ongoing dialogue becomes an ongoing debate. Jefferson is the most resonant figure in that debate because he straddles both sides of the argument with both eloquence and agility. Rather than tear down the Jefferson Memorial and thereby lose his tribute to human equality, my preference is to add the panel with his distressing words about racial inequality. Our dialogue will then contain a realistic reminder of what we are up against.

*One of the nation's leading scholars of American history, Joseph J. Ellis was awarded the Pulitzer Prize for* Founding Brothers: the Revolutionary Generation and the *National Book Award for* American Sphinx, a biography of Thomas Jefferson. *His book,* American Dialogue, *shows that the founding fathers worried about many of the issues confronting us now—corruption, foreign influence, and a divisive two party system.*

..................................................

# Why Activists Need Home

## By Jean Shinoda Bolen

A new generation of feminists is addressing the injustices they see at home—from domestic violence to inadequate food, water, and lack of housing—in every corner of the world. Over one million non-governmental organizations and grass roots organizations now focus on women's basic safety, while helping them to build strong families and sound regional economies.

In *Artemis: The Indomitable Spirit in Everywoman,* I show how the energy of an ancient Greek goddess has inspired this wave of global activism. In mythology, Artemis protected the young and vulnerable. Shortly after birth, she helped her mother deliver her twin brother Apollo. The herb that is named for her—Artemisia—has since been given to ease the pain of childbirth. In her temple, Artemis offered sanctuary to women and guidance to young girls. As goddess of the hunt, she spent many hours with her sisterhood of nymphs, exploring the marshes, the forests and the fields. And as goddess of the moon, she was attuned to the cycles of waxing and waning that govern the natural world.

Artemis was a virgin goddess, meaning that she remained one-in-herself, or psychologically independent. The quintessential tomboy, she was at ease with men, and every bit their equal in strength and skill. In our popular culture, the Artemis figure shows up in Disney's bow-wielding princess, Merida, in Katniss Everdeen of *The Hunger Games,* and in the fiery Dany in *Game of Thrones.*

We also see her in real life heroines on the evening news: in the courageous representatives of the #MeToo movement; in the work of Malala Yousafzai, a Pakistani teen who was shot for standing up to the Taliban and supporting the education of young girls; in Emma Gonzalez, a survivor of the mass shooting at a Florida high school, now working for tighter gun control; and in the young Swedish activist, Greta Thunberg, who has called world leaders to task for failing to combat climate change and protect our planetary home.

Artemis women are natural crusaders, fired by a fierce will to shelter and protect the vulnerable. They may live through tragedy and trauma, but they refuse to identify as victims. They stand up to bullies of all kinds, from perpetrators of rapes and domestic violence to oppressors of the poor and defenseless, to abusers of the environment. And they never give up. This is the new face of feminism.

Often the modern activist is formed by a challenging event at home. Between kindergarten and fourth grade, my family moved a lot. I was enrolled in seven different schools: in Los Angeles; Kew Gardens, New York; Black Foot, Idaho where children were bussed in from the reservation; Grand Junction and Denver, Colorado; and Monrovia, California. Then it was back to Los Angeles, where we settled down. In

United Nations terminology, we were "internally displaced refugees."

Though my grandparents came from Japan, my parents were born and educated in the United States. My father was a respected businessman, my mother a physician. We went on this odyssey to escape the evacuation and relocation of all people of Japanese ancestry to internment camps, where we would have been kept behind barbed wire, in tar-papered barracks in desolate places in the Western states.

Once out of California, we were again regarded as free American citizens. Our subsequent moves were necessitated in part by my father's efforts to get his parents and siblings out of the camps. While our country was at war, I enrolled in one school after another, often the only child with a Japanese face. This gave me a first-hand experience of social injustice and racism.

Families today are uprooted for many reasons, from economic recessions to famine, war, and climate change. During relocation, children have to cope with new schools and temporary housing. Such experiences support the development of an Artemis woman and have given rise to a new generation of activists and community leaders. We learn how to survive and thrive in difficult circumstances, vow to make daily lives better for others, helping people whose basic needs for home, security and sustenance have been ignored.

Instead of becoming victims, Artemis women seek justice and become even more determined to pursue their calling. They become role models and big sisters, and volunteer to rescue others. Early on I served as an advocate for women in the American Psychiatric Association and other professional organizations. My book, *The Millionth Circle:*

*How to Change Ourselves and The World,* inspired women who were active at the United Nations (UN) to form the Millionth Circle Initiative. I then became an advocate for a UN-sponsored 5th World Conference on Women (5WCW). Though we obtained the support of the Secretary-General and the President of the General Assembly, a UN resolution to proceed with this conference did not come to a vote. However, the idea gained momentum and international support through Women Economic Forum (WEF), the largest gathering of women entrepreneurs and leaders, worldwide. I had hoped that this conference would be held under the auspices of a joint WEF and 5WCW Mission Million 2022 in India, but that was not to be. When this gathering finally takes place, however, it will have been well worth the years of groundwork and perseverance.

Over the past four decades, I've done my share of public speaking, giving lectures and workshops in other countries. Though inspired and energized by these gatherings, I come home determined to clear the decks for a while, eager for some quiet time to write and reflect on my experiences. This is my way of balancing my psyche, making sure that my activism stays deeply grounded in my beliefs and honoring my own internal rhythms. As goddess of the moon, Artemis reminds us of the waxing and waning cycles we see in nature, and experience in our own biology. Her message is that extraverted time in the world must be followed by time-out for self-renewal and replenishment.

Intense involvement in a cause and an affinity for working with large groups are hallmarks of the Artemis-inspired activist. Though such a woman seems to have indefatigable energy and may inspire crowds, she also needs to tend to her personal relationships. Those close to her often wish she would show them the same commitment and constancy she reserves for her causes. Like wildlife in the forest, there can be a "now you see her, now you don't" elusiveness about an Artemis woman. She's so real and present, then she's gone for long stretches of work and adventure. That's why coming home is so important. An Artemis woman needs this time of grounding herself in the personal—of honoring her friends, her family, and her inner world.

In my books (especially *Goddesses in Everywoman, Gods in Everyman, Goddesses in Older Women, Crones Don't Whine*), I'm concerned with the way we balance our psychic energies and learn to draw on a wider range of human archetypes. I've found that an Artemis heroine is well served when she learns to honor the wisdom of Hestia, goddess of the hearth. Hestia's sacred fire was the center of the home, a source of heat and light, spiritual illumination, and daily nourishment. In contrast to the always-moving Artemis, Hestia is introverted, and content to be in the peaceful home that she creates.

Over my living room mantel, I've displayed a large painting of Hestia's ring of fire. On a table nearby are sculptures of wild animals, sacred to Artemis. This is an altar of sorts, where I honor my deep identification with the wildness at the heart of the world, my fierce need to go out into the world and champion the needs of others, and my need to sit by the hearth and simply be.

For the modern woman, this need to blend both Artemis and Hestia, the inner and the outer directed aspects of the personality, has led to an interesting trend. More and more of us are living on our own as a way to maintain this balance. In *Going Solo: The Extraordinary Rise and Surprising Appeal of Living Alone* (2012), Eric Klinenborg describes how living alone fosters a sense of personal control and self-realization and allows time and space for restorative solitude. According to the 2021 census, 37 million adults, or 28 percent of all Americans now live alone. This percentage has been steadily rising for the last 50 years.

Many women find living alone to be deeply soul satisfying. We can decide how to spend our time, whether to support a cause or be creative, when to keep our own hours and spend quality time with others. The rising number of younger women who are not marrying at all or marrying later in life, view this as the ultimate freedom, while many in the second half of life are delighted to be on their own, after years of living with parents, roommates, partners and children. In each case, home takes on a new meaning, as a place where we honor our own values and our contribution to the world at large.

Humanity is at a crossroads because we have consciousness and choice, and at the same time we are facing destruction of our planet by climate change, wars, and weapons of mass destruction. The beauty and ongoing life of the planet need to be protected—the mountains, forests, oceans, lakes and wildlife, from microbe to honeybee, salmon to polar bear, earthworm to eagle—all that lives instinctively and unconsciously in ecological interdependence. The Earth is sacred to Artemis—as is love for wildness in any form, and reverence for life.

Being an Artemis-inspired activist requires us to get out there and take on some heroic mission. But it also requires time out for reflection, and a deep sense of home.

Every woman who effectively marshals others to fight for a cause needs a sanctuary, a "room of one's own," where body and soul can be restored.

As we return from our demonstrations and our meetings and our marches, we need the grace of Hestia, the time to sit by the firelight and be at peace. That is the only thing that will allow us to sustain the gaze—to keep looking at what is broken then do our best to repair a portion of the world.

Here is some guided imagery for Hestia: Sit quietly for a while and invite Hestia into your meditation. Imagine there is a sacred fire glowing in the center of your chest, then let it spread throughout your body, bringing warmth and comfort. Take some slow deep breaths and let yourself surrender to the quiet. Once you are in a receptive, spacious state of mind, imagine yourself walking across a threshold into Hestia's presence. Look into her fire and be open to the images that come to you. Let your whole being relax and remember what it means to feel at home.

*Jean Shinoda Bolen, MD, is a psychiatrist, a Jungian analyst, activist, and author of 13 books that have been translated into over 100 foreign editions.*

PART IV

# HOMELY
# CONVERSATIONS

# CHAPTER SIXTEEN

......................................................

## Make Your Life Like Music

### With Helen Marlo

In our first conversation, Jungian analyst Helen Marlo explores the myth of work-life balance and how the rhythm of life changes drastically for new mothers. Her advice: Don't try to manage things with a flow chart. Make your life like music. Think of each day as a symphony moving from a crashing overture to a brief adagio then back to the up-tempo beat again.

Marlo is a Professor of Clinical Psychology and Dean of the School of Psychology at Notre Dame de Namur University in Silicon Valley and a Faculty Scholar with the Dorothy Stang Center for Social Justice and Community Engagement. A clinical psychologist and psychoanalyst in private practice in San Mateo, CA, she also founded Mentoring Mothers, providing emotional support for women from pregnancy through the birth process.

*We're going to talk about how the deck is stacked against working mothers and why. But I'd like to start with you. What's your first memory of getting short-changed as a mother?*

My doctor of obstetrics and gynecology is a man who has championed, supported, and cared for women his whole life. He is an amazing soul. As I was giving birth to my third child, he let my husband pull my daughter out, and the first thing he said as the baby emerged was, "Good job, Dad." It *was* a good job that my husband did. But I actually did a natural birth, with lots of blood and lots of work.

As a working mom, I notice that when husbands and partners do something supportive, people often say, "Oh my God you're so lucky." If a husband makes it to a child's school event, it's "What an amazing Dad!" If I'm late, I'm "an obsession career-driven woman."

***Was this lack of acknowledgement one of the reasons you started the organization called Mentoring Mothers?***

Yes, that and I wanted to address a new mother's general feeling of overwhelm—to give these women a place of connection and community. We meet with pregnant women at the local medical building twice a month to help them nurture one another. The idea is to create a more conscious experience of motherhood. Our goal is to support a woman's emotional and psychological development and assist her in becoming the kind of mother and the kind of woman she wants to be.

***What concerns do the women typically bring to you?***

Well, the comments I hear most often are these: "I just didn't think this would be so hard!"

"Nobody prepares you for what it is like once the baby comes out."

"Everything has changed. I just don't feel like myself anymore."

"I didn't think I would feel so exhausted, stressed, worried, and lonely."

"I don't feel bonded to my baby—some days I don't want to be around my child."

And finally, "I am afraid I'll repeat what I experienced as a child."

Women are concerned with issues of childcare, self-care, and family history. And of course, they are also trying to figure out whether and when to go back to work. There's not much support in our society for women who are trying to combine work and family.

***Do you think the two-paycheck marriage has put families under constant strain? Fathers are missing out because they're not getting enough time with their children and the women are just exhausted from trying to do it all.***

I see a lot of stress in one paycheck marriage, too. The significant thing is how the pay checks are negotiated. For women, this can be a status issue: "Oh my God, you poor thing, you have to work. Your husband doesn't provide for you." Or "You didn't marry well enough."

If the wife isn't working, the husband often resents the fact that he bears a greater proportion of financial burden. These husbands often think, "I'm really burnt out and having to work more and more and more because my wife would like to stay home."

***Many women calculate the amount of time they put in on the childcare and housework and feel they have to do more—based on how much less they are earning.***

Yes, yes exactly. When one paycheck is disproportionately greater, that triggers an unconscious conflict.

***Tell us what brings a woman into the consulting room and to see a psychologist and say, "I need help."***

Sometimes it's her physical health—fatigue or exhaustion. More often, she is experiencing an emotional overwhelm. A triggering of anxiety and depression, anger and resentment. Sometimes, there's the so-called "ghost in the nursery," something the woman lived out as a child that still troubles her—her own trauma, rage or neglect.

Often we end up recreating our childhood homes. Women may understand they have issues around their parents but there is something powerful in the trigger of home. That's why I developed Mentoring Mothers—to recognize the link between early home life and early trauma that gets cracked open with pregnancy and childbirth.

***Do you recall this case described by Donald Winnicott? He was treating a young boy whose parents were having trouble after the birth of the second child. The boy did not feel safe at home, so he took a ball of string and tied it around the legs of the sofa and then around the legs of the chair and the legs of the coffee table. This was his effort to bind the home together because his parents' relationship was insecure.***

The choices women make often mirror that fear of insecure attachment. A mother might say to me, "If I work more than four hours a day then I'm going to be neglecting my child. I was latchkey kid. I can't do that to my daughter."

Another might say, "My mom was a really smart and she resented having children because she never got to use her brain." Or in a similar vein, "Mother always looked good but she gave us no emotional warmth. I'm not going to repeat that pattern." These early childhood experiences affect the choices a woman makes when she has a family of her own.

They influence what kind of mother and homemaker she will choose to be.

*We don't seem to realize just how important home is in the formation of our inner lives. The Adverse Childhood Experiences Study showed that early trauma in the home leads to major illnesses later on. How do you see this in your practice?*

It plays out powerfully, and across the board. This was another reason why I started Mentoring Mothers. Look at the empirical studies about postpartum depression. Rarely do people think about this as post-traumatic stress disorder. Yet, a good 17 to 24 percent of women qualify for that diagnosis. They may have a number of symptoms, and they are not getting enough help.

*And if the memory of trauma is still uncovered, it can be triggered by the pregnancy?*

Yes, the experience of giving birth, and having a child to care for, can open up all sorts of memories and emotions.

*Is your goal then to get these women to a place where the home can ground them and provide a sense of sanctuary?*

When we can get them to that place, that's a real success. Part of my work is helping women realize how emotionally charged the topic of home is for them and what different meanings home has for them. The stay-at-home mom, afraid to leave her house, often has some early trauma to deal with. Conversely, there's the woman who can't bear to be at home and has to be out as much as possible. Our service focuses on helping these women to build a healthier connection to home than they had when they were growing up. Our goal is to facilitate a more flexible and more fully integrated relationship to home in all its dimensions.

***What's the importance of having downtime at home in the digital age?***

I see that as a much more important need of late. Today, we have more awareness of how much technology intrudes on the home space. And something as simple as developing our own rituals at home can be life-giving.

When my children were growing up, each received a magic box. We told them that the magicians came in the night and left this gift. The box might contain an encouraging message, or something concrete that they desired. The box also focused on relationships. It might contain a note, "This ticket is good for time with the family" or a photo of all of us together. We still have this ritual today. It's changed as the children have gotten older, but the magic box taught them that what happens at home is valuable, that there can be magic, there can be beauty—and a sense of delight in family life.

***Did you make each box to reflects the personality of the child?***

I did. One daughter has a box with purplish-blue marbled paper that contains photos of me when I was pregnant with her. The box is decorated with butterflies and flowers—symbols from a dream I had about her birth.

I incorporated another dream symbol into my son's box. The box is shaped like a boat and the top is covered in ribbons that look like a sail.

That ritual of receiving the magic box was really special for my children—even more so as they got older and learned who the magician was.

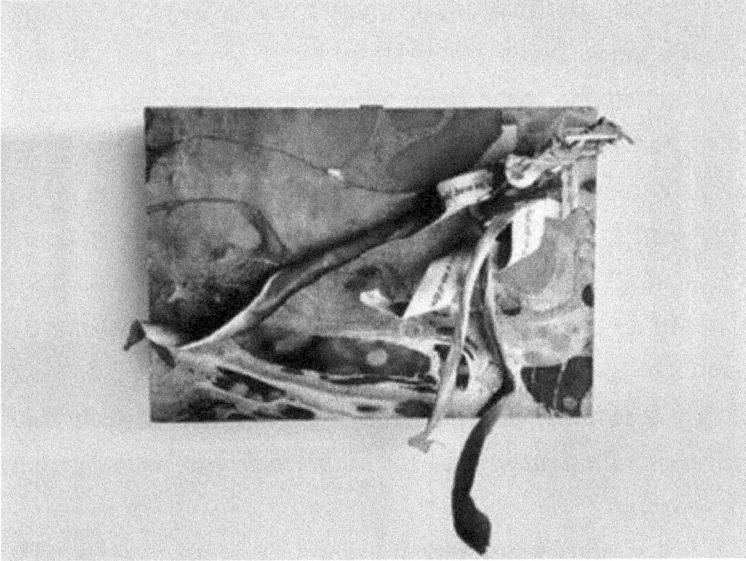

*The "magic box" Marlo created for her son*

***Can you talk about how you balance your work life
with time at home with your family?***

My father wisely said to me, "If you want to get
something done, give it to the busiest person you know."
I think he was talking not just about being productive and
getting a lot done, but about the value of having a full life.

I chose a profession that I loved. Not everyone does.
And then they are stuck and feel trapped. But I love what I
do and so I don't separate my work and family life so rigidly.

I have a very flexible schedule. I'm a night owl so I
go with my biorhythm and work late at night. This sometimes
makes my students laugh—"Oh, she sent me an email at 1:00
a.m."

I get to choose when I'm on the clock and when I'm
not. And the benefit is that I can spend a lot of time with my
kids.

I can be involved in their lives in ways that many career women aren't. I'm grateful that I can set my hours in my practice and that I have an academic job where I work on my own time-frame. When I teach weekend classes, my family comes up at lunchtime and we all have a meal together. This year, I was surprised by the number of female students who said, "You're modeling something for us when you have your family come for lunch." I just had them come because I wanted to see them!

*If you had to create your own magic box—one that represented a healthy and harmonious home—what would you put in it?*

I would like to have more time at home to relax with my family, doing activities we find fulfilling. It could just be sitting around the dinner table and laughing—without a cell phone or a computer in sight. Without any attempts at multitasking. Being able to have a good conversation is important.

Sometimes we push all the furniture out of the way, turn up the music, and have dance parties. We made our own disco ball in our living room and just plain have fun.

*Do you have any strategies to recommend for women who are trying to blend work and family?*

People often talk a lot about the importance of work-life balance, but I challenged that mindset when I was teaching wellness classes. I teach others to embrace a more fluid work-life rhythm and encourage a more responsive stance toward life. "This is the rhythm you're in right now, and it's going to end at a certain point. Then what will you do to replenish yourself?"

*That's a beautiful concept. One that's based on a sense of flow and of the fact that we live in cycles.*

Exactly, that's been a constructive approach for the women I work with. The concept of rhythm is much better than balance. Home is rhythm, I say, so make your life like music.

......................................................

# CHAPTER SEVENTEEN

# Aging at Home

## With Peggy Flynn

What's our history of aging at home? And how an we make home a creative stage set for the last part of life? These are questions I posed to Peggy Flynn, founder of The Good Death Institute and author of *The Caregiving Zone*. A graduate of the certificate program in Jungian Studies at the Chicago Institute, she is now a spiritual director, specializing in opportunities for growth in the evening of life. In this conversation, she considers the nuts and bolts of caregiving— and the importance of directing one's own story and feeling comfortable at home in one's final years.

***What changes to you see in the way we age today?***

One of the things I hear most often from older people is, "I want to age at home" or "They're going to carry me out of here, feet first." Well, that's not an issue any longer. For many people, nursing homes are not an option. They're very expensive, and as we speak, more and more of them are going out of business. So the reality is people will be aging at home, and they will be dying at home.

Home becomes independent living, then assisted living, then a nursing home, and eventually a hospice. That's the trajectory of aging, and we'll be needing to more and more services at home right until the very end.

*Before we talk about the life cycle in the home, can you explain how you came to this kind of work?*

Well, it wasn't something I put down as my ambition in my high school yearbook. It's been mostly evolved as people started coming to me for help. I kept finding myself in this situation with friends and neighbors and family, so it was really necessary to get some training and some skills.

*You write in The Caregiving Zone about your father showing up on your doorstep, and that sounds like what we call boot camp training in the topic.*

I'm the oldest girl in an Irish family, so I knew that whichever one of my parents went first, I would get to take care of the other one. I had this problem all worked out years before it happened. And I went through a whole process of considering the money and values involved in caregiving, and other issues like loyalty. So that when the situation manifested, I was ready. My father had surgery, he called me from the recovery room—how he remembered my phone number, I have no idea—and said, "I can't go through this by myself."

Because I knew what was going to be coming down the pike, I was prepared. So I was able to work with him. That caregiving stint was supposed to be six months, it ended up being three and a half years. So bootcamp lasted a long time.

Working with other families, I found that most of the trouble came because people weren't looking at the facts and facing up to their financial limitations. They wanted a Cadillac plan, but there was only enough money for a Volkswagen plan. How to tell the truth about what's possible right from the get-go is key. When people say, "Well, I don't want go to a nursing home." I often respond, "You can't afford a nursing home so take that option off the table." That takes all the emotion out of the discussion, then we can deal with the resources we have. Facing facts is a big thing. Families are often fact-free zones that run on distortion and wishes, wannabes, and if-onlys.

It all comes back to talking about home. What are the facts of home? And then addressing some real basic things such as the challenge of stairs, the danger of throw rugs, and whether the doorways are wide enough. Many people find focusing on that kind of detail challenging, but I find that relaxing.

***The caregiving zone is fraught emotionally. Siblings often argue over who's going to take care of Dad or Mom." And many older people don't want to admit that they need help.***

That's the big question: Can you get people there? All of a sudden, there is aging, illness, incapacitation—and this cannot be ignored. We're all experts in facing reality, but then we have to meet it head on. As the novelist Rita Mae Brown said, "Humans are volcanoes, spewing emotional debris through a rational crust." All that debris comes to the surface. And so one of the things I recommend is to bring in an outsider. Let a person who is not part of the family drama present the facts.

I also suggest applying American psychologist Abraham Maslow's hierarchy of needs: food, shelter, clothing, social, intellectual, heart, creativity, spirituality. What are the facts around those issues in this particular home?

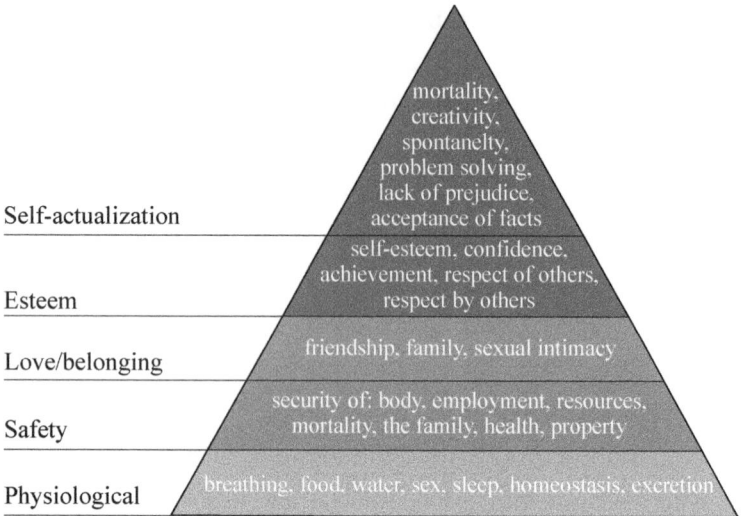

Self-actualization — mortality, creativity, spontanelty, problem solving, lack of prejudice, acceptance of facts

Esteem — self-esteem, confidence, achievement, respect of others, respect by others

Love/belonging — friendship, family, sexual intimacy

Safety — security of: body, employment, resources, mortality, the family, health, property

Physiological — breathing, food, water, sex, sleep, homeostasis, excretion

*Flynn has adapted Maslow's hierarchy of needs to the house---the bathroom is the place for hygiene, the kitchen for nourishment, the bedroom for rest, and the living room for socializing and a sense of community and belonging. In the evening of life, home becomes a stage set and each person a producer/director of the story of their own life.*

**When you counsel people on this hierarchy of needs, where do you usually begin?**

With the bathroom—that's where hygiene takes place and the bowel function is addressed. Is the bathroom safe? Is the bathroom adequate? You need to address the specifics: raised toilet seats, grab bars. Do you have things in the bathtub that prevent slippage? If the bathroom doesn't work, if the bathroom is not adequate, you've got a problem. If for example, the main bathroom is on the second floor, and someone can't navigate the stairs, that's an issue. So, that's the first thing to deal with.

The second thing I think about is the kitchen. Does everything in the kitchen work? Is everything accessible and reachable? Is the freezer big enough to hold enough meals?

***In the bedroom, what needs to be changed, or converted, or made more comfortable?***

Well, the bedroom is really interesting. Here we see the continuum of care in terms of equipment. For a long time, the existing bed—a single, double, whatever—will probably be fine. But as a person's need for care increases, they may need the convenience of a hospital bed with all of its adjustments. Or it may be time to move into a different room. If the bedroom is dark, or feels tucked away, people will often say, "I don't want to be stuck back there." So, at this point, maybe the living room gets converted into the bedroom.

***What do you do about a sense of beauty and attractiveness—to make sure the place reflects a client's personality and interests?***

A friend with a terminal diagnosis was very clear she did not want to die in her bedroom. She wanted to be in her living room. She had a beautiful craftsman house and so we went to the furniture store and bought a new sofa, because the one she had was inadequate for company. Now people could visit her and be comfortable, and she eventually died on that sofa.

We had fun shopping. Because she was a fiber arts person with a sense of texture, she knew what she wanted. She really got into the notion that she was creating a stage set. This sofa was her theater. There's a lot about aging that is theater, in the classic sense of the word. It's a drama. And so, when you have a drama, you think: stage set, costumes, props. My friend was very clear. She did not want to be surrounded by anything that looked medical. The sofa had a high enough back to hide all of her oxygen equipment. She could hold court from the sofa without appearing compromised. This was how she had lived her life, with elegance and grace, and this is how she wanted her last six weeks to be.

Illness, aging, dying is a drama. If you embrace it that way, then you can play with it, make a story out of it.

***You're raising the question, "What is this last phase of life going to be about? How can I make it creative, and communal, and still feel like I'm a part of life until the very moment when I'm not?"***

The only way you could do that is to accept your reality. To say, "This is what's happening." It's also important to know your values. For example, I am a fairly solitary person. And the worst thing for me to imagine is having all these people coming and going. This would not be my idea of a good time. This would not be in sync with how I live my life. I love peace and quiet. Other people who are very social, would not find that so appealing. So, it's one of those things I like to ask, "What do you like? How do you enjoy your life"?

The best thing you can do is consider all these things when you're well. I tell my clients, "Do it when you're in pretty good shape. Look at how other people have dealt with aging and dying and ask, 'Would I want that for myself?' Then begin to talk to people about how you want this time to look for you."

One client I worked with loved the composer Handel. My task in his last couple of weeks of his life was to deejay Handel. I set it up, so that whenever he was awake, he was listening to his favorite music. Other people came in and said, "We don't like that piece. Could we put something else on"? And I said, "No, this is what he wanted." That was my job, to make sure that even when he slipped into a coma, this man heard the music that he loved.

*How do you get people to view this transition creatively?*

I talk about the dark side of dying straight on. When it's denial, denial, denial, and there's no plan, everybody gets exhausted. And when no one will admit what's happening, one of the first casualties is good care for the person who's ill.

Sometimes the best way to care for the dying at home is to call a hospice service. You have access to a nurse and to trained home health people. Putting off that call means that as you're getting sicker and sicker, the people taking care of you are not well trained. I've known people who basically died from cancer taking Tylenol, because there was no one at the house who could prescribe the necessary pain medication. Denial can have very serious consequences.

I've also seen caregivers get injured, because they're trying to change the clothes of a person laying in a bed, or get them out of the bed, without a hospital bed that they can easily adjust. Or there can be a mishap because there isn't a commode in the room. So, there are consequences of denial for both those who are sick and dying, and the people around them. And a lot of that can be avoided if everybody sits down and says, "This is what's happening, so let's make a plan."

*Let's talk about how we've dealt with death in the past. Old Colonial houses used to have a dying room on the first floor—and a front door large enough to get the casket in. In those days, the wake was usually held in the dining room. And illness, death, and dying were a part of daily life.*

I think we are heading back in that direction—with more people dying at home. Tragically, though, there isn't

165

an extended family to support the dying process as there used to be. That's going to be our challenge. With that house you're describing, probably most of the family lived within 10 miles. There was an extended group supporting the one who was aging and dying, and then there were the three or four people—usually relatives—providing most of the care.

I think it's a very rude awakening when people realize, all of a sudden, "Oh, it's going to happen here. And hospice can only send someone to our home 12 hours a week."

***And what kind of stress does that place on caregivers and family members today?***

Sometimes families can't take it on. The term we use now is "the squeeze generation," for those with ill or aging parents. Usually these are women with children who are also working full-time jobs. Adding one more burden isn't realistic. It sounds very Norman Rockwell or The Waltons to say, "Okay, Dad, you can move in with us. We've got the space." But how could people know what kind of time it takes to provide personal care and regular meals for someone who is increasingly dependent? Often what seems like generosity can really blow up in the family's face.

It's very hard to say no, it's very hard. With my dad, I was very clear. I knew he and I could not live together, so I got him an apartment in the same building.

In some way, the dying part is the easy part. That last six weeks you can do on adrenalin. But it's the preceding years of increasing dependence that's a marathon. That means negotiating at every point that the situation of decline shifts to a new low.

I'll give you some examples—when it's time to stop driving; when stairs are no longer a possibility; when the person can no longer cook for themselves; when their cognitive decline makes the home unsafe for them, or others. You need to check in at all those markers and change a care plan accordingly.

In the best of situations, you can negotiate all that, but only if you're working with somebody who will negotiate with you in good faith. Often there isn't enough honesty between parents and children and that's a part of the stress. When dad says, "I can still drive—I'm fine" or, "There's nothing wrong with my memory. You just forgot to tell me that." or "I don't need hearing aids—if you just would stop mumbling."

Those are the kinds of issues the care-giving generation is going to come up against, and it's better to have those conversations when everybody's well.

Many of us will be doing peer caregiving for our friends our own age, and that's a whole different negotiation—easier in some ways, and harder in others.

*One women's group I know of has made a pact: the members will tell each other when they start repeating themselves and to give each other honest feedback.*

Yes, but this phase of life is also about learning how to receive care, learning how to accept help. That's a whole new skill set. As a caregiver, I'd give myself an A but in receiving care, I'd give myself a C. It's a challenge to receive, it's a challenge to be dependent, so what I say to people is, "Practice being dependent before you actually are dependent."

*A friend's mother recently entered a nursing home and had a bumpy time. Now she has settled in and continually thanks her caregivers. She's in a place of total gratitude, and often says, "Thank you so much for taking care of me."*

If this happens, and it comes from an authentic place, then everyone is blessed.

I think that this kind of gratitude is something we can all start working on today. Last week, I was taking the bus to a meeting, and the stop was three-quarters of a block away. The wind chill factor was 21 degrees, and I waved frantically to the bus driver as she headed to the stop. She pulled up right next to me. I thanked her very much because if she'd kept on going, I would have been left standing there for 10 minutes or more, feeling the cold wind coming off Lake Michigan. I think that the practice of living in gratitude gives you resilience—then when things are really hard, you are more able to adapt.

When I was in college, I was earning money on the side by doing home care in the country in Santa Cruz, California. On this four-mile stretch of road, I had four clients, all elderly women, living alone in their houses. I was often the only person they saw from one the week to the next. They were just holding on and their loneliness was palpable, like a second person in the room. I asked one of the women, who was more approachable, "All of you live on this road … What if you moved in together?" And she said what every one of them felt, "I cannot have another woman in my kitchen."

When I got home, I realized, "Boy, that's me too." And I thought, "Okay, Peg, from now on, you are going to invite other women into your kitchen." Suddenly this room shifted from, "my kitchen," to "the kitchen." That's what I mean when I talk about looking at your resistances, then making an effort to expand your boundaries. It's all about recognizing where and how you need to change.

***You're saying that if we come into the evening of life with the right attitude, then everything shifts.***

I often think of what Jung said, "Thoroughly unprepared, we take the step into the afternoon of life; worse still, we take this step with the false assumption that our truths and ideals will serve us as hitherto. But we cannot live the afternoon of life according to the program of life's morning; for what was great in the morning will be little at evening, and what in the morning was true will at evening have become a lie"[22] So how do we enter this new period, and how can we do so consciously?

First of all, we have to remember that we need other people, and that it's our job to make it easier for people to be around us. That's important. Another key factor is the willingness to be pleased.

I had a client in her 90s who was in cognitive decline. Her daughter had a hard time being at the hospital with her for a lot of reasons—mostly because she just loved her mother so much, it tore her up inside to see her like that. And so we had an agreement that if Alma had to go to the hospital, I would go with her.

At one point, I was at the hospital and the doctor came in and asked, "Now, who are you?" And I said, "I'm a friend of the family and a friend of Alma's." And so he turned to Alma and asked, "Is it okay that she's here? Do you know who this is?" Alma looked at him with her clear blue eyes and said, "I don't know who she is anymore, but every time I need her, she comes."

We built that relationship over the years, and every time she needed me, I showed up. There was a bond. Though she didn't know who I was, she was happy I was there.

Now I want to come back to the notion of how we manage when we are at home. We are creatures of home. Home is everything. A good question to ask yourself is, "What are the five basic elements that make home a home for me?" This is not the same for everybody. And then, you must be able to communicate that to others.

When I was training home health workers, one of the things we learned was that caregivers brought their own food, which was often very different from the food the person they were tending had around. Then, the aging person would feel, "Well, this isn't my house." Why? Because it no longer smells like their house.

Sense of smell is the oldest sense for a mammal. When the little creature is born, it's got to find the nipple, right? It's got to find the milk. It does so by smell—that's the only sense we're born with fully formed.

One of the things I suggest for caregivers, is to keep apple pies in the freezer. If a person gets agitated, put a pie in the oven. The house will be filled with a scent that will immediately calm them.

When I was doing end-stage care, sometimes I would meet a person in the last few days of their lives. Maybe they could communicate and maybe they couldn't. One of the things I did was to look in their kitchen, then at their bookcases and at their music collection. That would tell me a lot about what home meant for them. I wouldn't bring something in that wouldn't fit in with those values.

One of the things I recommend to people who are growing older is this. Tell people, "If I lose my marbles, here's my music; here's what I like to eat; here's what will just be very agitating for me, and very, very disruptive; and here's what will comfort me."

One psychologist I work with says, "Equanimity is in direct proportion to our ability to feel comfort." Well, in the aging process, equanimity is in direct proportion to others' ability to comfort us, so we need to tell them how to do that.

One time, I went to a man's house and he was totally freaked out, almost in tears. I asked, "What's the matter?" And he said, "My worst nightmare was that I would get sick and lose my mind. Well, I'm losing my mind, I cannot find anything. And I think I put something some place and then it's not there."

I said, "First of all, I know you, you're not losing your mind. Something else is going on here. Are you on any new meds?" He said, "No, no, no." So, I suggested, "Walk me through your house." He pointed to his things and said, "I didn't move this!"

It turned out that four different home care people had been there. All were people who loved him, but they did things their own way. They would do the laundry, do the dishes, go to the store, and then they would put things back where they would normally put things in their own house. They'd fold the clothes like they usually do. They would put the groceries where they would have stored them. So, I said, "Let's go through your apartment and put these things where *you* want them. Then, I left notes for the caregivers, "Please follow these instructions exactly."

***To preserve another person's sanity, you have to follow their domestic routine.***

Yes, we all have our accustomed ways. And that's an old-fashioned term. It means caring enough for another person that you go into their place and observe how they do things.

Again, we come back to this notion of a stage. If we look at the person we are trying to care for as the producer/director, then we are going to take our cues from them. But if we come in there and our attitude is, "I'm here to save you" and "I'm here to show you the error of your ways," that's not going to be helpful. Do you know why this attitude is so bad?

*If you do that, you're running your own hero's journey, and it has nothing to do with the person who's looking for home and sanctuary.*

Exactly! Caregiving is not a hero's journey. It's not. The person who's dealing with their end-of-life issues is on the hero's journey. So, the question is: are you there to support them as their story unfolds, or are you there to usurp it and have your own drama?

Another thing to remember is this: consciousness has nothing to do with cognition—those are two different things. That's why the story about Alma is so important. Her cognition was shot, but her conscious awareness was flourishing. She knew that we were in relationship. She knew what she was feeling. And even though she was in a hospital bed, she felt at home.

I keep coming back to this: there's home in your body; there's home in your environment; there is home in your relationship network. Home is bedrock. And it's not just that for humans—it's the same for all living creatures.

CHAPTER EIGHTEEN

..................................................

# The Art of Living in Uncertain Times

## With James Hollis

We are living in an era of transition, morally and socially, and many of us feel that we are no longer in control of daily life. How can we cope with this period of chaos and reorganization? How is adversity calling us to stretch and grow?

Analyst James Hollis, who taught humanities for 26 years before becoming a Jungian analyst, says that literature can help us navigate uncertainty, and feel more at home within ourselves. Hollis lives and works in Washington, DC, and is the author of 20 books on depth psychology;his most recent are *Living Between Worlds: Finding Personal Resilience in Changing Times* and *A Life of Meaning: Relocating Your Center of Spiritual Gravity.*

In this conversation, Hollis considers what great writers—from Sophocles to Shakespeare—teach us about the benefits of enforced solitude. He also examines Jung's advice on ways to counteract the stress of modern life and find our inner home.

*America has been dealing with a pandemic, an economic downswing, long-standing problems of racism and social injustice and climate change. How can we feel at home in a radically changing world?*

You're talking about how the current crises in our culture have called into question all the answers that we thought we had about life. Actually, that's a pretty good thing. It's disconcerting to ego consciousness, of course, because it undermines our sense of security and our sense of control. But we need to be questioning our relation to the environment. We need to be questioning our relationship to minorities. We need to be questioning our institutions and our political system. I always think questions are better than answers, and underneath all of these is really a summons to a larger accountability.

I have this question, "Is America going to grow up and be accountable for its history, be accountable for its economic policies, and be accountable for the vast divisions that lie between so many of our people?" I see this as an enormous invitation and a threatening invitation. But perhaps history is making it necessary.

The truth is, the moments where we grew the most were moments of conflict, perhaps of loss, even crisis, and perhaps, of suffering. There's an old medieval saying that suffering is the fastest horse to completion—not that we want it or invite it. I think, in our own time, the bankruptcy of the all the things you've mentioned—our materialism, hedonism, narcissism—is patently obvious. That leads us to questions like, "What abides amidst all of these changes?" So, I consider this a healthy shakeup, albeit an uncomfortable one, in which people are invited to consider what really matters to them.

*In your book, Living Between Worlds, you say that literature can help us cope with uncertainty and fear. How?*

Literature represents an effort to explore what's going on inside a person from the beginning. In a sense, artists and writers were the first psychologists. They engage the images that emerge from their own depths and dialogue with them, whether it's in painting, or music, or writing, producing some kind of conversations that allows us to gain access to what's going on inside us.

As Jung said, he was swarming with the materials of the unconscious in his own midlife crisis. Until he could grab hold of an image from the depths, he couldn't dialogue with it, couldn't make it conscious. The image was the key, the point of entry, the aperture, into some understanding of what was going on inside him. And so it is with all of the great arts and in particular, literature.

*How do you think literature gives us a better understanding of our changing times?*

If you want to know what's happening in today's headlines, you can read the scriptures or the Greek tragedies— or the myths of ancient peoples. Human nature has not changed at all. Technologies change, social practices have changed, and values have changed, but the human psyche is very much the same. If you really want to know what's going on in the unconscious, you should examine myths. Again, myth is a tangible expression of the energies that are rising from within. So many things that happen in our time seem shocking, but they shouldn't be, if one is a student of history.

*You make Sophocles come alive as you focus on Antigone. I'm wondering what message her story has for us today.*

As you recall, she was caught between loyalty to her brother, her family, and the gods, and her loyalty to the state. When her brother rebels against the established order, as embodied by King Creon, he is killed. Antigone, understandably, wants to bury him with the appropriate rites, when, in fact, he's considered an enemy of the state. She's told, in a sense, "You have to choose what your highest value is." Those are painful and difficult choices, and as we know, she pays with her life.

*This reminds me of the mothers in Portland putting their bodies and their lives on the line for Black Lives Matter. There was very strong sense of Antigone's presence—when we saw these women demonstrating on the evening news.*

I've been deeply moved by that. They're also bearing witness to the fact that sometimes you have to stand up for a value and you have to pay a price. If you're not willing to do that, it's not much of a value—or maybe you're not much of a person.

*I want to turn next to Hamlet. You talk about him as a man who's stuck between "fight or flight." How do we experience that emotional paralysis today?*

Well, it's been argued that Hamlet is the first truly modern character in Western literature. Hamlet is faced with a dilemma. He is summoned by the Danish state and by his own morality to avenge his father's murder. On the other hand, he's struggling with forces within that he doesn't fully understand. The reason Hamlet is so modern is that he knows, "I am my own problem." In the opening of Act III, Hamlet says, "And thus the native hue of resolution is sicklied o'er with the pale cast of thought and loses the name of action."

Now, that's a perfect description of a complex. We have an intention, but something invisible reaches up and shuts us down. We all have stuck places. And times where to move forward causes an unacceptable level of anxiety that has the power to veto forward motion. Hamlet understands that he can't appeal to others, he can't appeal to the gods, he has to figure it out for himself. In the end he has to push through his dilemma and act.

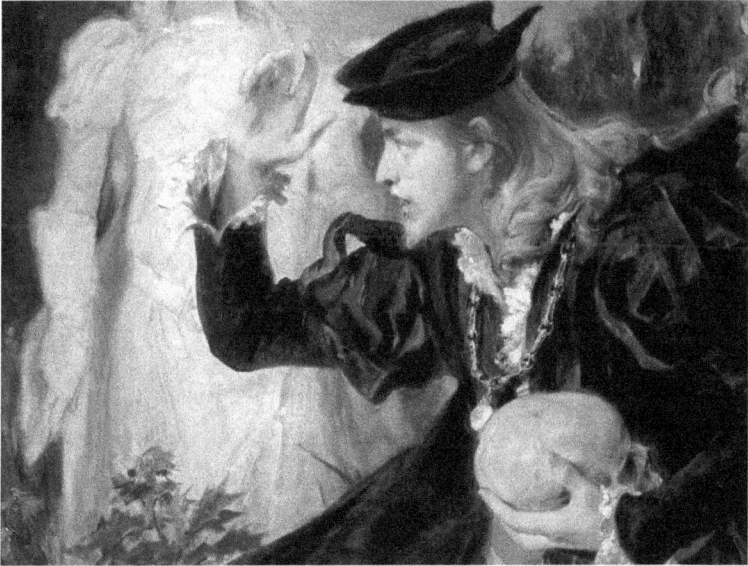

*By Pedro Américo - Visão de Hamlet.jpg, Public Domain,*
*https://commons.wikimedia.org/w/index.php?curid=22937131*

Antigone is caught between two outer value systems. But Hamlet is caught between two dueling complexes. He's been the subject of many psychological treatises through the years. Ernest Jones, one of Freud's disciples, wrote a very interesting book on *Hamlet and Oedipus*, but that's a story in itself.

Hamlet is a predecessor to the modern individual, who says, "I know what I need to do, but for reasons I don't understand, I can't do it." And we all have that issue within us.

*I'm wondering how that's playing out in the wake of the pandemic. Many experience some form of psychic numbing or personal exhaustion. An inner voice seems to be saying, "Wait and see what happens next before you act."*

I think the pandemic was the first time in American experience since World War II that every household, and every single individual on this continent, was facing some form of threat. Now, we've had other national events, like the disaster of the 1986 Space Shuttle Challenger or the attack on the World Trade Center in 2001, but for many people, it is that thing that happened "out there." COVID touched everyone, and it had life or death consequences.

This has been a real call to awareness. What we've seen is an elusive enemy who slips away from all of our assumptions, along with the bankruptcy of our system. And rather than being the world leader in this time, we have managed things very poorly. I think the pandemic has been an occasion for people reframing their sense of self and world and reframing our national story, as well. All of these experiences we're talking about are humbling to the American culture, and that's a good thing. Because there's a little too much rah-rah and too little accountability for what really does not work in our country.

The other piece of that, of course, is enforced isolation. I've just finished eight hours of analysis with folks, and the number-one topic for the last five months has been, as you might well expect, the difficulty of coping with economic worries and feelings of boredom and listlessness, drift and malaise, floating depressions and so forth. I think more and more Americans are being invited to a conversation with their own souls and finding that this is not necessarily a comfortable relationship. Ours is a culture that prides itself on its distractions, and a lot of those distractions like sports events and picnics and family reunions and travel, are now constricted. So, folks have had to find their own resources. A large number of people, however, have found new sources of creativity and interests.

*It's almost like we've gone back into a pre-digital age in terms of solitude.*

There's an old saying that the cure for loneliness is solitude. In solitude, you are present to yourself, and therefore you're never wholly alone. The real question is posed by Jung. He felt that we need to find out what supports us when nothing supports us. A lot of people found that their work schedule, their busyness at the office, and what I call their "plug-ins" to family and friends and other activities— once those are removed, that energy inverts as a depression. Now, what are you going do with it? That's the key. Can you tolerate being with yourself?

*A lot of this has to do with the smallness of daily life. T.S. Eliot addressed that theme in The Love Song of J. Alfred Prufrock. A man longs for meaning yet his life is measured out in coffee spoons.*

Most men have lost contact with their souls a long time ago and, trust me, I spend a lot of time in those conversations. I put it this way, in talking with women's groups.

Imagine three things. First of all, cut away your friends, the people you really share your intimate life with, your thoughts about your marriage, your children, your body, your worries. Those people are out of your life forever. Second, sever your link to whatever you consider your guidance center, call it your instinct, your intuition, whatever. And third, accept that your worth as a person will depend largely on your proving your productivity and meeting certain abstract standards or goals set by total strangers.

*That is such a painful description.*

Well, that's the point. Women have said, "Oh my God, that's awful. How horribly lonely." The truth is that's the plight of 90% of men. Even while surrounded by loving families.

*In our high-tech age, we tend to forget about men who work with their hands. Are we losing respect for men who fix, repair, and build things?*

I agree that we have been overvaluing the abstract thinking function. We've moved predominantly into education and healthcare, which are important, and of course, data processing. And where does that leave the work of hands and the essential dignity of the person digging the ditch or working in the coal mine?

My grandfather died in a coal mine as an immigrant. He had no choice in life but to take the only job he could get, but you're right, the work of hands is part of how we connect to nature, to each other. It's part of how people serve their culture, their families.

*And it's how they care for their homes. I think that's what Jung experienced at Bollingen, working in stone and building the tower at his country retreat.*

That's right. The tower he built was without electricity, and he lived there deliberately as a 14th-century person with candlelight. He would get water from a well and that sort of thing. He actually hated the telephone and said, "Notice what a tyrant it is." You can be involved in meditation or in the deepest conversation with a person, the tyrant rings, and there you go. As Rilke noted at the beginning of the last century, the world we've created is not much of a home for us.

*Are there any psychological insights that might help us navigate this era?*

We become prisoners of that to which we are attached, that's the paradox.

Jung said encounters with the Self are usually felt as a defeat for the ego. What does that mean? The ego is a necessary thing —we need it to interface with the external world, but it's also a little tyrant. And it wishes to have what it wants when it wants it. That's where materialism, hedonism, and narcissism come in. How do I entertain myself and make my life pleasant? These are not federal crimes, but our assumption that this is the goal of life makes it harder for people to age, and harder for them to deal with change and loss.

The German word for serenity is *gelassenheit*, and it means the condition of letting go.

*What ideas do you think we need to be brave enough to relinquish?*

One of the chief American fantasies is that we're supposed to be happy. I have nothing against happiness, but happiness as a goal ultimately trivializes a person's life. Happiness is a momentary experience of being in right relationship to your own soul. When you're doing what is truly right for your soul, not necessarily for the world around you, you're flooded with that feeling. Happiness arises out of the strangest situations.

For example, I don't enjoy being a therapist and listening to people's suffering, hour after hour, but I find it profoundly meaningful. I can't imagine doing anything else. So, I would say meaning is worth committing your life to because it has staying power. When it doesn't, then move on and find out what does, because that is a sure way to be in relationship with your own soul.

*The root of the word "suffer" also means to allow. If we don't allow ourselves to contemplate the death of our culture, or our individual lifestyle, how can we move forward in a meaningful way?*

The ego will never be thrilled with death, but on the other hand, as Wallace Stevens said in his poem, *Sunday Morning*, "Death is the mother of beauty." It makes us appreciate things that are transient, it provides our life with meaning. If we weren't mortal, we'd be like the idle rich, where there's nothing more to do, except kill time.

*I'm wondering if the unconscious doesn't call us to account by posing an enormous problem for each generation. My grandparents lived through the first world war and the 1918 flu epidemic, and my parents through the Great Depression, another world war, and the birth of the atomic bomb.*

My parents, too, went through the Depression and the war and anyone who did was profoundly changed, and I think, in a good way, humbled by it. They didn't take certain things for granted because they realized how provisional and how contingent they really were. I do think we as Americans have ridden high in the saddle for a long time and haven't had to feel accountable for the world and for our own values because there's always tomorrow.

There's something to be said for optimism, at the same time, a naive optimism means you ignore the reality of the world around you, so the world has to come to us, and surprise, surprise! What has not been faced inwardly, as Jung pointed out, will tend to spill into the world, and in some way, we played a role in it.

*I'm curious what books you're reading now to find your own compass, your own sense of home?*

I'm starting the Hillary Mantel's three volumes on Thomas More and Henry VIII. That's a formidable mountain to climb, but I believe it's going to be valuable —because what we see, in different garb, is the timelessness of the human psyche.

The power of reading is something that I learned as a child. I grew up in impoverished circumstances, and my parents were really crushed by the Depression and lack of education. My father was pulled out of eighth grade and sent to work for the rest of his life. For me, teachers and books were my heroes, because they opened points of entry into a larger world. They showed me there are things to see and to explore out there and I remain deeply grateful to all of them.

*If you had to give a reason for optimism as we go through this period of major change what would you say?*

I don't think anyone knows about the future. The new organizing images will arise from the unconscious.

If they don't, then frankly, we're going to be at the mercy of images created in laboratories and by computerized programs and so forth. The better hope for the future lies in the core resilience of the human spirit.

If we do what is right for us, something inside of us supports us. We have elemental systems that nature has given us, and we knew this as children. But because we were tiny, vulnerable, and dependent, we had to turn them off to adapt. That includes the feeling function. We don't choose our feelings, but feelings are a qualitative analysis of how our life is going. We can reject our feelings, anesthetize them, and ignore them, but they tell us something. And feelings occur before our thoughts occur about them.

Secondly, we have our own energy systems. When you're doing what's right for you, the energy is there, you feel that flow. So in a sense, the key to what really is important is pursuing what energizes you.

Thirdly, we have dreams that are commenting upon our lives on a daily basis. I'm in my 80s now, and if you live to age 80, you will have spent six full years of your life dreaming. Think of that! That's an extraordinary amount of activity in the psyche. Nature doesn't waste energy. I think part of that activity is assimilating the magnitude of data and stimuli that come to us on a daily basis, but another part is our own larger self-reflecting upon our life. If you pay attention, dreaming can be a profoundly meaningful engagement.

Fourthly, and most important, is a sense of meaning which is unique to each of us. You can't trade yours for somebody else's meaning. You have to find what your life is asking of you and engage in some kind of conversation. I've often said to people in therapy, "This is not about pathology, this is a deepening conversation around the meaning of your life's journey, and it will be the most interesting conversation you'll have in your whole lifetime. Moreover, out of that comes the quality of your relationship to other people."

There's a paradox here: No relationship, whether it's an intimate relationship or a relationship with a whole group of people, can be any more evolved than my relation to myself. So where I'm stuck, my relations will be stuck.

***Well, you're talking about being stewards of our own psyches and learning to feel more at home in our own skin. But we can also be better stewards of the culture.***

That's right. Again, thinking about the sequestering experience, many people have been invited to that in a new way because they don't have the distractions. Blaise Pascal said in the 17th century that the chief problem for humanity is people's inability to sit by themselves for very long in their own private chambers. If I can't tolerate myself, how can I tolerate someone else?

We all know too, what I want to deplore in myself, or I want to deny in myself, I'll be looking for in my neighbor. That's an old idea, the projection of my shadow onto others.

Another element to our divisiveness, though, is that there have been major dislocations and changes in our economic structures, and many people feel—and I have deep sympathy for this—that the future does not include them.

On the other hand, I also understand that all of us, to some degree, might say we want things to change, but when change comes, it unsettles the ego's security agenda. So, the future belongs to those who can move with those changes.

***Any other advice for how to feel more at home within ourselves?***

The first half of life, we all have to deal with the question, "What does the world want of me? Can I develop enough ego strength and resources to deal with it?" The second half poses a different question, and that is, "What does the soul want of me? What wants to come *through me* into the world?" That's not about being comfortable, that's not about fitting in, it's about serving something that makes your life worth the journey. If we don't do that, somehow that whole journey gets sabotaged on behalf of fitting in or comforting the ego.

Jung put it this way. He said, in effect, that our job is not to fit in; it's to be eccentric. If you fit in too easily, you have had to hone away the edges, the things that make you unique. I'm not talking about an adolescent rebellion—seeing your peculiarities brings a richness back into the world. Living them is the adventure.

# CHAPTER NINTEEN

## Homecoming from Homer
to the Wizard of Oz

### With Phil Cousineau

In this conversation, award-winning writer, filmmaker, travel guide and storyteller Phil Cousineau talks about the joys and challenges of homecoming—one of the oldest themes in the world, repeated from *The Odyssey* to *The Wizard of Oz*. Cousineau's fascination with other cultures has taken him from his native Michigan to Marrakesh and from Iceland to the Amazon. He's written more than 40 books, including *The Hero's Journey, Stoking the Creative Fires, The Art of Pilgrimage, The Book of Roads,* and *The Lost Notebooks of Sisyphus.* For ten years, he was host of Global Spirit, the first "internal travel series," on PBS and LINK TV.

*I'd like to begin by asking why we're so preoccupied with homecoming here in America.*

Great question. My friend Pico Iyer, the travel writer, told me recently that there are more refugees than any time in human history. There is a constant population of people wandering, leaving home, searching, making us more rootless than ever before. That's a global issue. But Americans, from the very beginning, have been rootless. And right now we're

187

engaged in a big debate: Who belongs here, who can really call it home? Who gets to stay?

I travel a great deal and I often hear from my European friends who think it's a little curious that so many Americans go to Europe to find their roots. Now, why would we do this? Because on some level, we still don't feel quite at home in America or like we even could be.

*What you're saying is important—that as a nation, we don't feel at home.*

Yes. What did Will Durant say in *The Lessons of History*? It took England 700 years to produce Shakespeare and France 900 years to produce Voltaire. Like that, it takes centuries to come up with a common identity.

As an athlete and sports follower and someone who's written a book on the history of the Olympics, I find it curious that we have used the verb "to root" to describe our relationship with our sporting teams for at least 150 years. I don't think that's an accident of language. I think it's telling us is that when we root, root, root for the San Francisco Giants, or the Manchester soccer team, we are sinking roots because we identify with them.

*Our teams are our mascots for a sense of place. When there's a home game, there's all of this spirit that's palpable in the stadium.*

It's almost obsessive. We wear the colors, the caps, we wear the jerseys. We deeply identify sometimes to the point of going berserk. But James Hillman, the great American depth psychologist, said that rather than try to suppress that, we should actually *increase* the pageantry. We are talking about our pride in the home team, the pride of the team that we root for.

I just came back from Detroit where I grew up. Many people were walking around with sweatshirts with what they call "the old English D" for the Detroit Tigers, while others wore DIA shirts from the Detroit Institute of Arts. Now, what does this mean? It means that Detroiters are *sinking roots,* which is necessary for a rebirth, a renaissance of a city. They are doing so by identifying not just with sports, but with culture, history, the *genius loci,* spirit of the place. And they are doing so with a new sense of pride. Why? Because for about 25 years or so, it's been very hard to identify with a place that went from one of the fastest growing cities in the world—two million people in the 1960s—to a shell of its former glory. Detroit had about 630,000 residents at last count. This is the most precipitous decline in population in urban history.

It's very hard to begin to rebuild without a sense of pride. People who don't love or identify with where they live will burn the place down, let it decay, out of sheer despair. How we feel about a place cannot be underestimated in any discussion about home or homecoming.

If you're ashamed of home, which is traditionally a sanctuary, a kind of archetypal anger builds up. If you're not proud of your home, if you aren't happy to go back there. If you don't find a sense of sanctuary and safety, you will, consciously or unconsciously, undermine the place you live.

### *What do you think has turned Detroit around?*

"Economics," like "ecology," is a word with home at the center of it. It's based on the old Greek *oikos*. So, economics is at root a love of home. To turn Detroit around took time, money, and love. It took a couple of major tech companies and some banks. Real estate was extraordinarily, almost egregiously cheap for a time. Then, investment came and pride followed and then, the people themselves decided to defend and remake their idea of home.

*I have read about a strong homesteading movement in Detroit. People are reclaiming these crumbling brownstones, putting in sweat equity—redoing the plumbing, the walls and the floors. This movement is drawing a younger generation, who want to live in a big city, but can't find one they can afford. And so, they're flocking to Detroit, saying, "This is a place we can build with our hands."*

Yes, that's true. I returned there a few years ago because of a film I worked on about our home baseball park called *Stealing Home*. How about that for turn of phrase? The very first run that was ever scored was at Tiger Stadium with Ty Cobb, stealing home. But the city wanted to tear down that historic stadium.

We showed the film, which later got nominated for an Emmy. After a screening at the Detroit Public Library, I walked the neighborhood—a long neglected wasteland—looking at all the little businesses cropping up Woodward Avenue. New shops had been opened and the area had attracted a whole flock of young Lithuanians, Latvians, Russians. Why? While the property was very cheap. I kept hearing something really beautiful: "This is where the edge is this." A 25-year-old said, "New York is behind us. I would get swallowed up in Los Angeles. But here I can make a contribution." Now, isn't that how you build a home?

*This is perhaps the true meaning of home—that it gives you space to grow.*

On that trip, I kept hearing people say, "I want to bring this city back." In other words, "I want to build a home." You know Greek myths as well as I do. There's this wonderful notion of Hestia, who's the goddess of the hearth. But, Hestia was not just about the individual home. There was a Hestia sanctuary in every town, every city, with 300 major cities in ancient Greece. That's what I'm alluding to, that there is something sacred about our home turf. I think it's important to remind ourselves to look beyond the economic aspect of a house. The equity, the mortgage and so on. There's also a sacred element. And the sacred element is what you will fight for and it's what you build a family around.

Going back to the Greeks, I love this idea of *xenia—a* code of hospitality. We reference that in our language now when we talk about its negative side, *xenophobia*, or shutting people out—the hatred or the suspicion of strangers. But, the Greeks have another beautiful word, which I would like to bring back, *xenophilia*, or the love of strangers, expressed in generosity and hospitality. In practice, it means reaching out to them, "Would you like to come in for some tea? Or maybe have some dinner?" Many scholars believe this was one of the keys to the Greek miracle, a belief that we are all strangers looking for home, so let us treat each other well. Xenophilia is about making visitors feel at home.

***You've written a lot about pilgrimage, what it means to go away from home in order to find it again.***

Let's consider the Australian walkabout, the Aborigine walkabout as a pilgrimage. Going back to the site of the ancestors to be replenished, to have a vision. I think that happens right up to the modern day. The pilgrimage is the journey that you can't *not* take. I love the double negative in there. In other words, there is a crisis, and your husband or wife can't save you. Your best friend isn't going to give you the answer. Your rabbi or your priest can't help you. Nor can your psychoanalyst, who you've been talking to for ten years. But, there is something deep in the human soul; I call it the psychotropic function—I don't mean taking drugs, I'm talking about the turning of the soul, the turning of the psyche.

***You went back to Greece and tracked the steps of Odysseus coming home to Ithaka this summer. So tell me, what turn did this story take?***

I've been going to Greece since 1975, but Ithaka is very difficult to get to so I didn't actually visit Odysseus' island until recently. Now, I'm about to lead a tour there, "In the Footsteps of Odysseus and Penelope." My approach nowadays is to include the recent and powerful new interpretations brought to us by female scholars around the world. So, I will be telling both sides of the story in this tour, giving voice to the women and the goddesses. This way we can talk about the hero and the heroine's journey.

This story has been in us for about twenty-seven hundred years, probably longer, if you go back to the oral tradition. So why is it important now?

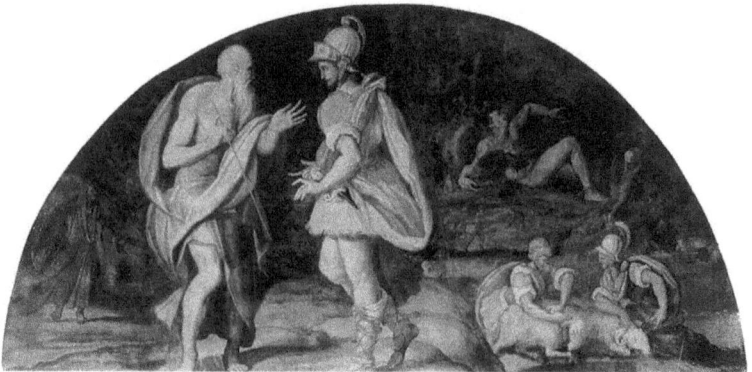

*Alessandro Allori, courtesy of WikiMedia Commons.*
*Odysseus questions the seer Tiresias.*

Odysseus reluctantly goes off to war and as he leaves, he's trying to take care of business. He's just become a father. He has an infant son. So he turns to his best friend Mentor, and essentially asks, Will you take care of my son while I'm away? That figure is the origin of our word *mentor*. He is the person who tends to the young when others go off to war.

Odysseus fights for ten years before Troy is brought to its knees and then razed to the ground. It takes him ten years to get from the west coast of what is now Turkey back to the west coast of Greece. My old friend Joseph Campbell, the great scholar of mythology, once joked that he had to earn his way back home. To do that, he had to overcome, or learn to deal with, two things: monsters and women.

This is the awakening of a man who has not quite appreciated his wife, Penelope. And he has upset the gods. Now Poseidon is wreaking havoc on his effort to get home again. In other words, *he has to earn his way back home*. This is part of the genius of this book.

One of the most compelling parts of the story is when Odysseus becomes lovers with Circe. She offers him immortality, saying in essence, "Just stay with me. You will be immortal. We will make love forever. You will never want for anything." But Odysseus is pining for Ithaka. He is feeling what has come to be called nostalgia.

"Nostalgia" comes from *nostoi,* the stories of coming home, and *algia,* pain. It refers to a bittersweet experience. It's not sentimental. Odysseus is pining for Penelope, for his son Telemachus, and the land. So Circe tells him, "There's only one person who can help you get home again because you have offended the gods—and that's Tiresias. You have to go down to the land of the dead and talk to him."

For me, this is one of the most magnificent aspects of Homer's book. The hero must descend into the underworld to find Tiresias, the sage. Now, here's the psychological revelation: The soothsayer says: You can get home again. But you will have to suffer.

It is not easy to get home again. The gods will make it difficult for you to do this. This message slays me: You will have to curb your desires and the desires of the men in your crew. In other words, it's your own desires that keep you from getting home again.

And then, what do we do when we get back home? We can revert right back to the whole cult of distraction and desire. And we will still be lonely if we don't sink our roots into where we are.

How can we accomplish that? By knowing the history of the place, the music, the people who lived there before us. By paying attention to the smells. When was the last time any of us walked around our neighborhood and didn't touch our cellphones, but instead just picked up a scent? I live in North Beach here in San Francisco. I can walk around the neighborhood passing bakeries and coffee shops. My sense of smell is often what brings me home again. Smell is the strongest and the most transportive—the most mythic—of our senses.

### *So how does this help us?*

Smell is a way for us to go home again. A single smell of castor oil takes me there; Grandma Dora used to pinch my nose and pour castor oil down my throat and say, "Someday, you'll thank me for this, Philip."

Well, what has happened? Suddenly my Grandma Dora is standing right here in the room with me. I suggest that if we are trying to get home, we revisit it with our senses.

Here's another example: Late last night, my wife Jo and I went to hear a magnificent musician, Georgios Xylouris, who hails from Crete. The room was filled with two hundred people, two thirds of them Greek. Why were they there listening to Cretan music in San Francisco? They were there to go home again through music, to let the sound transport them. You could hear the gasps during this concert as listeners were taken back to Crete, and were probably thinking about parents, old loves, the boyfriends and girlfriends of their youth. Our sense memories strengthen our connection with home.

*That would be a wonderful writing exercise: What do you see when you look out your window? What do you smell when you step out into the street? What do you eat that brings back memories of home? How does it feel to polish the furniture, to care for things in your own house, to touch them, to get a sense of their own aliveness?*

When James Joyce wrote *Ulysses* (we know this because we can see in his journals and diaries), every chapter was associated with a mineral, a god, a smell, a sense of touch. He said he wanted to baffle scholars for a thousand years. Yet, here's the clue. By reading *Ulysses*, scholars can reassemble Dublin brick by brick.

I think that's the key for getting home as well. Using all your senses.

*Let's talk about The Wizard of Oz—a contemporary coming of age story about a young person losing and then re-finding home.*

In November 1956, CBS television aired the film to great acclaim. Within a few years, the telecast became an annual tradition, especially around Christmas and Easter, and somehow helped bring families together around the virtual fireplace of the television. Now, what's the overlap? The theme of rebirth or resurrection. In a true hero's or heroine's journey, the character dies symbolically at the beginning and is reborn by coming home again.

There's the very last scene of the movie. Dorothy is lying in her bed, feeling her head because she's had a big bump. And she's wondering, "Where am I?" And the good witch Glenda says, "If you just wake up, you will see that you have always been at home."

To me, that's the key to the film. It's metaphysical, which is very unusual for a Hollywood film. What was the essence of Buddha's teaching? Wake up! Most great spiritual teachers have the same message. We go to sleep, as Gurdjieff put it. And then philosophy, religion, travel, art begin to wake us up again. What that means is this. If you wake up, and all five senses are alive, you realize you can be home *anywhere*.

*At the start of the story, Dorothy has lost her parents and she's being raised by Auntie Em. And she likely has that feeling, "Do they really love me? Is this really my home?"*

The theme of abandonment abounds in traditional fairy tales, as Bruno Bettelheim showed us in *The Uses of Enchantment*. But Frank Baum felt we can no longer rely on European fairy tales. So he decided to make one for American children.

How did he do that? Toto is a reminder that you need to get back to your animal nature. You can't get along with ratiocination. You can't get by on a superhuman intellectual effort. You need contact with the natural world. Baum also knows it's lonely to be a kid. It's lonely to be in that never-never land in between youth and adulthood. But, if you find allies—the Cowardly Lion, the Tin Man, and the Scarecrow—that helps. If young people can find allies, they will not feel alone.

Yes, that's the formula throughout human history. What about the classic and corrosive American loneliness? Our myth of individualism? We are the greatest innovators and tinkerers in human history, from Thomas Edison to Steve Jobs. However, the myth of individualism pits us against our own families, against the community, against the tribe. In *The Wizard of Oz*, we see young Dorothy, alone—scathingly alone. But then, she finds three allies. When they take the Yellow Brick Road into the Land of Oz, they skip and dance. They sing, they exult. It's one of the most enchanting moments in movie history. I think that's how we all feel when we find we're not alone.

***That skipping, that lightheartedness. The joy of discovery. These, too, are elements of homecoming.***

The Russian artist Chagall once said, "I paint in order to be surprised." I believe that the greatest writing also happens when we surprise ourselves. "Where did that come from? How did how do you think of that?" I like to think about the surprise of coming home again, and bringing a gift to the people you love.

***That gift is in sharing the nature of our own experience.***

Yes. When I went back to Detroit, was it the same? Was I the same? No. That place is almost completely different. But, so am I.

*Is there a particular ritual you perform when you get back from your travels?*

I put on some blues or some classical, and when I hear my music, I feel like I'm home here in San Francisco. That's what grounds me.

I do think there's a universal need for a homecoming ritual. For millennia, when a pilgrim came back from his travels, the neighbors and the family would put on a fête or feast. You didn't just sit around and think about what happened in your six months of being on the road. You got reincorporated into the community. People danced and they sang and they ate together. So, you break bread. You have a drink. You clink glasses. Those are all elemental rituals, where you say,: "All right. That part of my life is over for now. I'm home again."

*Is there something special you do with your wife and son once you arrive home?*

We tell stories. My son Jack is 23 and we have a kind of traditional greeting upon my return. "So, Pop, was it fun? What did you do? Who did you meet? What did you see?" Those are elemental questions. My inspiration for this is Chaucer's *Canterbury Tales*. The pub owner at the Tabard Inn in London advises the pilgrims heading to Canterbury to find a stranger on the first day of travel to tell their story to: "I am from England. This is who I am. This is what I do." Then, Chaucer follows that with another psychologically deft suggestion. On the way back, you have to tell another stranger what happened once you reached Canterbury Cathedral. He knows that it is important to describe how your pilgrimage has changed you, as your depart for home.

This story was written about eight hundred years ago but, psychologically, it is so astute. The moment we begin to talk about the journey. "This is who I saw. This is what I felt"—we incorporate our travels and bring our experience home.

So, what did I tell my son when I returned from Detroit? "Jack, I saw many people. I was honored at the library and on my way there, I had a wonderful writers' retreat at the James Thurber house in Columbus, Ohio. But, the most moving element of my journey was that I went to the grave of your grandfather." I could see my son was deeply moved by that. It's a bit of a risk sometimes to tell our friends and family what was truly the most important part of our travels. But, you know what? I cannot have a complete trip back home without going to my father's grave and going out to raise a glass with my old friends.

# CHAPTER TWENTY

......................................................

# Finding Our Home in the Cosmos

## With Brian Swimme

Physicist Brian Swimme likes to talk about finding our home in the body of the universe—noting that the cells in our bodies, and the dust on our bookshelves, originated with the Big Bang. A professor at the California Institute of Integral Studies, he is author of *The Hidden Heart of the Cosmos,* which describes in vivid detail how the universe, and life as we know it, came into being. But, he's more than a scientist. He's a storyteller—describing with a sense of awe and wonder, how humans fit into this galaxy, this solar system.

Swimme is the author of *The Universe is a Green Dragon*, coauthor of *The Universe Story* with Thomas Berry, and producer of the DVD series: *Canticle to the Cosmos*, *The Earth's Imagination*, and *The Powers of the Universe*. He also created the Emmy award-winning film and book, *Journey of the Universe,* drawing on discoveries in astronomy, geology, biology and the humanities.

*As a scientist, how do you define the word "home?"*

I like to think of the Milky Way galaxy as my home— here we are on Earth, on our little cozy planet. But, once we know that the Milky Way galaxy as a whole gave birth to our stellar system, then the Milky Way created the sun, and the earth comes out of the sun, we begin to realize the roots of our existence. The Milky Way is our home. This is what gave birth to us.

*Is part of the reason that we don't think of this larger home because we are so deprived of looking at a natural sky? Today, so much interferes with our direct perception of the universe.*

Well, that of course is the great sadness. I live in the San Francisco Bay area and it has blotted out the universe for its habitants. On a good night, in the past, an indigenous person would have seen 3,000 to 4,000 stars. Now, that experience is almost impossible if you're living in a city. In San Francisco, when you look up, you can see 30 stars. There are 3,000 to 4,000 wanting to peak through but they can't get through the pollution.

*Today, we pinpoint where we are on Google maps and yet we don't know where we stand in the body of creation.*

And yet, we do. We have the makings of a new creation myth, and this is what I've devoted my life to. We now have direct empirical evidence that around 14 billion years ago the universe was very small, small as a walnut, and very simple, just consisting of elementary particles. Over those 14 billion years that the universe has been developing, it brought forth stars, galaxies, planets and butterflies and skyscrapers, and we find ourselves inside an amazing creative story.

*As small as a walnut in the beginning. How do we get from something so tiny to something so vast?*

At present, the universe consists of around two trillion galaxies. Each galaxy having around 100 billion stars. No human up until now knew this. The big question was: Is there one galaxy or are there many?

Now we have this sense of this vast universe, and we know that it came from a very, very small space. You ask how can something the size of a walnut give birth to two trillion galaxies? I can give you the scientific theory. But, I want us to remain in the state of awe that we have actually located the birth of the universe. That's the great thing about our new creation myth, it just shatters our preconceptions about the nature of existence.

The most startling discovery, I think, in all of modern science is this expansion of the universe. But, the second most startling discovery is the realization that elementary particles are emerging into existence out of emptiness. The term in science is the quantum field, and this is the primary reality. The quantum field doesn't *have* things, it simply is a realm that *gives birth to things*. This generative realm pervades the universe. All the particles that seem so solid, and that for so long we thought were eternal—they're not! They're momentary excitations of the quantum field. That means everything we look at is like a flame.

### How does this impact human life?

Let me give you an example of a discovery in contemporary cosmology that has kind of amazing implications for social theory. I just talked about two trillion galaxies, that they're all expanding away from each other. And this expansion is strange.

This simplest way of saying that is this. When we look at the universe from the Milky Way galaxy, we're looking at the other galaxies out there as well. They all appear to be moving away from us, and from that, we conclude that we are at the center of this expansion.

But here's the kicker, if we found ourselves at another galaxy far, far out in the universe, we would think the same thing—that all galaxies are expanding from that point. So, we're in a very weird situation that's very different from what we thought. The truth is this: Every point is the center of the universe. This goes against the thinking of the modern era, where we believe we can arrive at a single perspective and see the truth!

Our perspective might be based on what's good for America, on Communism, or Darwinism or Christianity. But now we're discovering that all of those perspectives have something to offer. We're even questioning the notion that the human is the ultimate species, that our point of view is what really matters. From this new orientation, every species is central to the web of life.

And I think that, as this understanding seeps into our social theory, we will realize that every culture, every race, every civilization has value, and we will be living in a very different world than we are right now.

*You've also pointed out that we have a direct line back to the Big Bang in the dust that's under our beds and on our bookshelves. We're talking about a kind of primal material that's always existed since the beginning of the universe, right?*

We are. All of the hydrogen atoms of our body come from a time almost 14 billion years ago. Each of us has been assembled by the universe. Each of us. The hydrogen atoms come from the very, very beginning. And then, later on, the stars explode, and they give birth to calcium atoms and phosphorous atoms. Our cells still have the same dynamics of those early cells, so each of us is a 14-billion-year construction.

The Misminay Indians in South America say, "In order to be human, one must dwell upon the immensities of the universe." I just love that. You don't just have to be an adult with a job, with credit cards, no. You have to dwell in the immensities of the universe because that is your larger self. This insight has been cherished by indigenous groups for millennia. We're discovering it anew in the scientific context.

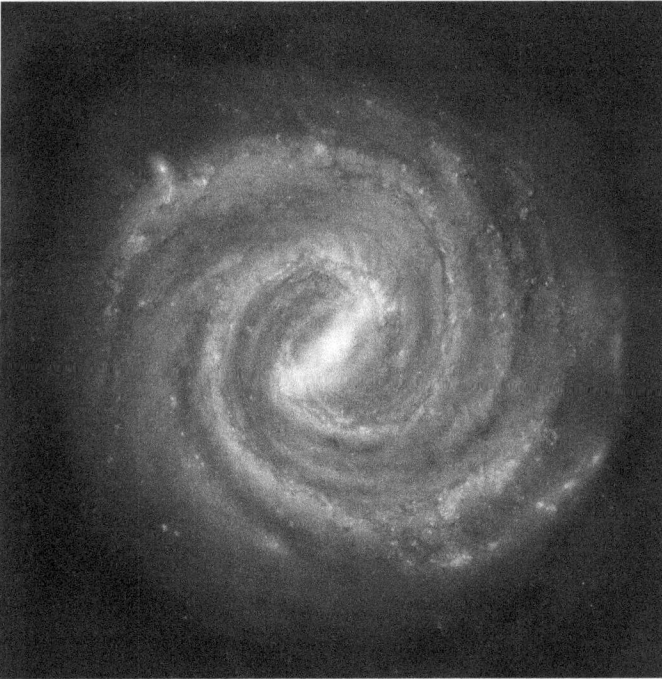

*Nick Risinger - Own work Adapted from NASA images: 236084main MilkyWay-full-annotated.jpg Messier51 sRGB.jpg*

***For most of human history, the dominant belief has been pan-psychism, the sense that everything is alive and has a presence. As we focus on the miracle of creation, will we begin to have an I-Thou relationship with the material world?***

That's a great statement. An I-Thou relationship, yes.

Let me give you a response from mathematical cosmology. One of the true mysteries we've touched upon in science has to do with the way in which the universe is expanding. The simplest way of saying it is this: If the universe were altered, even slightly, in its rate of expansion, there would never have been the structure as we see about us now. It's almost impossible to believe, but this is coming from the work of Stephen Hawking. He was the first to calculate that if you altered the expansion even by one part in a trillion, then there wouldn't be this amazing universe we live in today. That means then, that a planet like Earth was aimed at by the dynamics of the early universe.

When I think about that I quiver because, in science, we never talk about the universe having direction. But that's starting to break down.

***You mean we're beginning to think about intention?***

That is exactly what I'm saying. I'm saying that there's a form of intention we can even call *cosmic* intention. I'm saying that the universe intended stars, intended life, intended what we see about us and that includes boulders. I got this huge charge when I first learned this from Stephen Hawking. I realized that a rock is intended by the universe—that it's a cosmological construction.

This universe was going to make sure that rocks and boulders and life came fluttering forth and that is a step toward regarding each peg in the universe, as sacred or holy or something of that order.

***This sounds like the pre-Socratic philosophers with emphasis on the sacredness of earth, air, water, and fire.***

Absolutely. I remember when I first came across Pythagoras who talked about the music of the spheres, and that phrase did something to me at a deep level. I never got over it. Some way or another, I knew that Pythagoras, and the others, were in touch with something that can easily escape the reach of mathematical science.

***Is that why you set your film, The Journey of The Universe, on Samos, the island where Pythagoras was born?***

Absolutely. I think we live in an era that's something like that of the pre-Socratics. We need bold new intuitions about the nature of the universe, not just coming from science but coming from human intuition. This is one of the great statements by Thomas Berry—that we need to reinvent the humans at the species level. It's not just about creating a new economic system, or new religion, or new type of education. We need to reinvent ourselves as cosmological beings, to come alive with the sense of awe and the glory and the grandeur of our existence.

***What is the role of chaos in cosmic evolution?***

That's a difficult topic for us to consider because we fear destruction and we fear our own annihilation. One of the things that has struck me is the way in which the universe *relies* upon destruction, it relies upon chaos. Just to give you an example: When we examine particles coming forth from the quantum field, we see that they come apart in pairs. And so, a proton will come forth with an anti-proton. And when they meet, they both annihilate each other. Our current understanding is that there was this huge upsurge of particles, but a slight asymmetry set in. For every billion anti-protons, there were a billion-plus-one protons. So, right from the beginning, there's this massive annihilation with only one proton squeaking through.

Let me just give one more example to tie it in. It was a big shock for biologists to discover that over the course of three-and-a-half billion years of life, at least 99% of the species that came forth have gone extinct. So you think, "Whoa, the species that we see now are less than 1% of the number of species that originally came forth." This is the universe we have to deal with. It creates all these forms of life, and then it destroys them. And so, annihilation and creativity go together.

There's no way we are going to eliminate chaos or disruption or annihilation. The universe thrives on death. It's absolutely essential to the ongoing creativity of the universe.

### *How do we grasp this on a personal level?*

The question I ask is, what aspects of my life should be annihilated? Or another way of saying is this, what parts of my psychology are actually blocking my own creative development? And this is the way then to enter consciously into the annihilation process of the universe, because what happens with these vast annihilations is that new life comes forth and its life that has novel features.

Just to sum it up, the universe hates to be bored. The universe is deeply committed to bringing forth something new and interesting. And so, that's how at least I look at this terrible dynamic of chaos and destruction. It's part of what is needed for the universe to show a form of beauty that has not yet manifested.

We need a framework of consciousness to understand the remarkable time that we're living through.

*What really fascinates me about this explanation is that plus-one proton. All these protons and anti-protons keep cancelling each other out, and then the plus-one just skips through. If we can identify with the plus-one that makes it through the we can believe in positive change. We have a reason to believe that what we do, might count.*

To be part of that plus-one proton that makes it through the fence. Yes. I like it. That's what we can do.

*How can we help children feel more at home in the universe?*

When my wife was teaching kindergarten, she asked me to come in and talk to the students. When I'm teaching adults, I point out the ways in which Newtonian science and classical physics have been replaced by quantum theory and relativity, and all the rest of it. Obviously, these kids weren't going to know anything about that, and so I started to tell them how the universe grew up from a seed. Then, I focused on how the stars created the atoms of our body. And then, the stars dispersed throughout the Milky Galaxy and then here we are. And I said, "Each of these atoms actually came from a star."

A little kid in the first row was looking up at me as I was talking and didn't move his eyes away from mine. Then, he lifted his hands up and touched his cheek. It was so fantastic. He was entering into his participation in the universe and recognizing that he was a cosmological being.

I think we need to become better storytellers. These young minds, they're prepared. They're ready to hear the truth. They already know, in an intuitive way, that the galaxy is their home, and their bodies came from the stars.

# Endnotes

[1] "C.G. Jung: A Personal Memoir," by Elizabeth Osterman, The Elizabeth Osterman Archives at the C.G. Jung Institute in San Francisco.

[2] Jung, 1989, pp. 125-126.

[3] Jung, 1989, pp. 158-159.

[4] Durrell, 1969, p. 158.

[5] Hunt, 1989, p.104.

[6] American Journal of Preventive Medicine, 2015, pp. 245-258.

[7] De Botton, 2008, p. 107.

[8] De Botton, 2008, p. 107.

[9] Americans Must Say "No" Interview with Carl Jung in 1931 for The Sun, a New York newspaper published from 1833 - 1950. (Jung, 1977, pp. 48-49).

[10] Weber, 1916, p. 32.

[11] On Jung's relation to his kitchen utensils, Ruth Bailey writes, "You should visit it [Bollingen]. I have helped Jung perform some rites there. In the morning, when he came into his little kitchen, Jung would greet each one of his cooking utensils-the saucepans, pots, and frying pans. He told me I must also do so. "They understand and appreciate it." Jung always used the same frying pan and pots because they were his friends, and he considered them old acquaintances with whom to chat in the solitude of his retreat. For Jung, all things are animated with their own life, or with the life he transmits to them! ~Ruth Bailey (Serrano, 1997, p. 98). "As you know, in olden times the ancestral souls lived in pots in the kitchen." (Jung, 1973, p. 168).

[12] Jung, 1989, p. 225.

[13] Jung, 1989, p 236.

[14] Noël, 2023.

[15] Jung, 1967, para. 114.

[16] Jung, 1967, para. 114.

[17] Cope, 2015, p. 168.

[18] A transcript of Krista Tippett's interview with John O'Donohue, February 28, 2008, transcription can be found online at https://onbeing.org/programs/john-odonohue-the-inner-landscape-of-beauty/.

[19] Personal communication, Betty Sue Flowers.

[20] Personal communication, Jules Cashford.

[21] Hillman, 1998, p 54.

[22] Jung, 1969, para. 784.

# References

*American Journal of Preventive Medicine* (2015). *Vol. 14.*

Cope, S. (2015). *The Great Work of Your Life: A Guide for the Journey to Your True Calling.* Bantam.

De Botton, A. (2006). *The Architecture of Happiness.* Pantheon.

Durrell, L. (1969). *Spirit of Place.* Dutton.

Hillman, J. (1998). *Inter Views: Conversations with and Laura Pozzo on Psychotherapy.* Spring Publications.

Hunt, G. (1989). *Honey for a Child's Heart: The Imaginative Use of Books in Family Life.* Zondervan.

Jung, C.G. (1961/1989). *Memories, Dreams, Reflections.* Recorded and edited by Aniela Jaffe. Vintage Books.

Jung, C.G. (1967). *Collected Works,* vol. 7. Princeton University Press.

Jung, C.G. (1969). *Collected Works,* vol. 8. Princeton University Press.

Jung, C.G., Hull, R.F.C. (Trans.) (1973). *Letters,* vol. I, Princeton University Press.

McGuire, W., Hull, R.F.C. (Eds.) (1977). *C.G. Jung Speaking: Interviews and Encounters.* Princeton University Press.

Noël, M. (2023). *"Morale," in "Le rosaire des joies" from the anthology, Poésie Gallimard.* Translated from the French by Phil Cousineau and published in the document, *Parcours Façades,* by Vincent Adelus.

Osterman, E. *C.G. Jung: A Personal Memoir*, The Elizabeth Osterman Archives at the C.G. Jung Institute in San Francisco.

Serrano, M. (1997). *C.G. Jung and Hermann Hesse: A record of two friendships.* Daimon.

Weber, M. (1916). *Essays on Art.* William Edwin Rudge.

# Recommended Reading

**Introduction**
*Memories, Dreams, Reflections* by C.G. Jung

**Chapter One: The Poetry of Place**
*Anneliese's House* by Lou Andreas-Salomé, English translation by Raleigh Whitinger and Frank Beck

**Chapter Two: Typology at Home**
*To Live in the World as Ourselves: Self-Discovery and Better Relationships Through Jung's Typology* by Sally V. Keil

**Chapter Three: The Mythology of the Man Cave**
*A Home for the Soul: A Guide for Dwelling with Spirit and Imagination* by Anthony Lawlor
*The Temple in the House: Finding the Sacred in Everyday Architecture* by Anthony Lawlor

**Chapter Four: Renovating with a Shaman**
*Sea Glass: A Jungian Analyst's Exploration of Suffering and Individuation* by Gilda Frantz

**Chapter Five: Far from the Irish Sea**
*At Home in the World: Sounds and Symmetries of Belonging* by John Hill

**Chapter Six: American Icarus**
*American Icarus: Reflections on the Absent Father* by
Pythia Peay

**Chapter Seven: These Wilds Beyond our Fences**
*These Wilds Beyond Our Fences: Letters to My Daughter on
Humanity's Search for Home* by Bayo Akomolafe

**Chapter Eight: The Dance of Exile**
*The Great Work of Your Life* by Stephen Cope

**Chapter Nine: Coming Home to the V.A.**
*Madness: In the Trenches of America's Troubled Department
of Veterans Affairs* by Andrea Plate

**Chapter Ten: Pandemic Dreams—Horrors or Healers?**
*Pandemic Dreams* by Dierdre Barrett
*Trauma and Dreams, Robert Jay Lifton and Oliver Sacks* et al.
*The Earth Has a Soul: C.G. Jung on Nature, Technology and
Modern Life* edited by Meredith Sabini
*A Little Course in Dreams* by Robert Bosnak
*Tracks in the Wilderness of Dreaming* by Robert Bosnak
*Creative Imagination in Medicine, Art and Travel,* by Robert
Bosnak

**Chapter Eleven: What Myth Now?**
Anselm Kiefer's Breaking of the Vessels
https://publicdelivery.org/anselm-kiefer-vessels/
"The Culture Complex and Addiction to Dominion: Psychic
Evolution Cannot Be Thwarted" by Jerome Bernstein in
*Cultural Complexes and the Soul of America*

*Myth, Psyche, and Politics* edited by Thomas Singer
"Cultural Stories and Media Story Telling" by Betty Sue Flowers in *The Reality of Fragmentation and The Yearning for Healing: Jungian Perspectives on Democracy, Power, and Illusion in Contemporary Politics* https://aras.org/sites/default/files/docs/014Flowers.pdf

**Chapter Twelve: From Active Imagination to Wildlife Activism**
*Dream Animals* by James Hillman and Margo McLean (illustrator)
*Animal Presences: Uniform Edition of the Writings of James Hillman, Vol. 9*
*Voyage of the Turtle* by Carl Safina
*Song for the Blue Ocean* by Carl Safina

**Chapter Thirteen: Grasslands Woman**
*The Way of the Wild Soul Woman* by Mary Reynolds Thompson
*Reclaiming the Wild Soul* by Mary Reynolds Thompson

**Chapter Fourteen: Dialogue on the Mall**
*American Dialogue: The Founders and Us* by Joseph J. Ellis

**Chapter Fifteen: Why Activists Need Home**
*Artemis: The Indomitable Spirit in Everywoman* by Jean Shinoda Bolen
*Goddesses in Everywoman* by Jean Shinoda Bolen

**Chapter Sixteen: Make Your Life Like Music**
*Motherhood: Facing and Finding Yourself* by Lisa Marchiano
*Mothering Without a Map: The Search for the Good Mother Within* by Kathryn Black

**Chapter Seventeen: Aging at Home**
*The Caregiving Zone* by Peggy Flynn

**Chapter Eighteen: The Art of Living in Uncertain Times**
*A Life of Meaning: Relocating Your Center of Spiritual Gravity* by James Hollis
*Living Between Worlds: Finding Personal Resilience in Changing Times* by James Hollis

**Chapter Nineteen: Homecoming from Homer to the Wizard of Oz**
*Once and Future Myths* by Phil Cousineau
*The Lost Notebooks of Sisyphus* by Phil Cousineau

**Chapter Twenty: Finding Our Home in the Cosmos**
*Cosmogenesis: An Unveiling of the Expanding Universe* by Brian Swimme
*Journey of the Universe* by Brian Thomas Swimme and Mary Evelyn Tucker
*The Dream of the Earth* by Thomas Berry

9 781685 032180